TOTAL BREATHING

TOTAL BREATHING

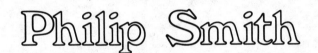

Illustrations by Doug Rosenthal

McGRAW-HILL BOOK COMPANY

New York ▪ St. Louis ▪ San Francisco ▪ Bogotá
Düsseldorf ▪ Madrid ▪ Mexico ▪ Montreal
Panama ▪ Paris ▪ São Paulo ▪ Tokyo ▪ Toronto

1 2 3 4 5 6 7 8 9 S M S M 8 7 6 5 4 3 2 1 0

First McGraw-Hill Paperback edition, 1980

LIBRARY OF CONGRESS CATALOGING IN PUBLICATION DATA

Smith, Philip
  Total breathing.
  1. Breathing exercises. I. Title.
RA782.S59   613'.192   79-26994
ISBN 0-07-058989-5

Book design by ROBERTA REZK

FOR POP
my favorite breath of inspiration

CONTENTS

PREFACE

DURING ONE OF MY frequent visits
to Miami, I broke my foot while running and was confined
first to bed and then to crutches for six weeks. As an active
person, I did not look forward to this period of rest and
recuperation. I thought it would force me to be almost
completely inactive. In an effort to maintain some level of
fitness, I recalled the effects of breathing from my yoga and
martial-arts training. In both of these disciplines, the breath is
used as the fuel with which to power and enhance the body.
I began to breathe in a controlled fashion for hours at a time.
Using the breath to exercise my chest and strenghten my
stomach muscles, I found that I could also ease moments of
pain.

Fascinated, I began researching the various ways in
which people used their breathing to accomplish goals in a
wide variety of activities—from acting and singing and sports
to Tai Chi and Kundalini and meditation. In my reading I
came across accounts of past civilizations that had developed
entire cultures around the practice of controlled breathing.
Both the ancient Egyptians and the Hindus felt that breathing
provided the basic energy for all forms of life.

In particular, the discipline called Kundalini, practiced
by master yogis, promised its practitioners total
enlightenment as well as complete control over the workings
of the body through the mastery of breathing. The doctrines
of yoga stated that life was measured not by the number of
years, but by the number of breaths one was allotted in a
lifetime. By slowing down their rate of breathing, yogis
reportedly could greatly enhance their lifespan. A true master
could make a single breath last for several hours.

Of course all these fantastic achievements required a
lifetime of singleminded devotion. What interested me was
the idea of finding a practical system of breathing that was
applicable to our daily lives. It seemed so important and so
obviously a vital component in our pursuit of physical fitness
and mental tranquility. Whether one is jogging or playing
tennis or meditating, breathing plays a crucial role. The more
I looked and read, the more I realized that breathing was the

missing connection for the integration and control of body and mind.

I spoke with several friends in the medical profession who agreed that the importance of breathing to our overall well-being is often largely ignored. After all, it is oxygen rather than food or water that keeps us alive from minute to minute. It is the air we breathe that helps fire the neurons in our brain, fuel the workings of our cells, and provide the basic life force that keeps us going. They expressed a great deal of interest in the possible applications of breathing to sports, stress reduction, and general good health.

I began to develop several basic breathing exercises that seemed to help both myself and my friends with increased energy and an overall feeling of vitality. By being aware of my breathing throughout the day, I watched how it changed in myself and in others under various conditions—while running, before sleep, under tension, and while working. In general, most people breathe in a shallow manner, often hardly breathing at all. The value of any breathing exercise seemed to be in its use of the respiratory system to its maximum potential, to get as much vital oxygen into the body as possible while at the same time removing as much waste carbon dioxide as possible.

More and more friends were sharing with me the ways in which they used the breath for greater endurance, vitality, and stress management. It became clear that an understanding of the use of the breath was an important aspect of everybody's training program as well as a continual source of energy and relaxation. Many persons might feel that they have no need for instruction in proper breathing. What they fail to realize is that even though one always breathes automatically, the breath is a valuable tool that, with conscious training, can provide important benefits for the body and mind.

It is quite amazing how a simple process such as breathing can affect so many of the voluntary and involuntary functions of the body. It is my hope that you will make *Total Breathing* a lifelong practice that is both enjoyable and endlessly beneficial.

PHILIP SMITH

New York
January, 1980

TOTAL BREATHING

ABOUT
BREATHING

BECAUSE WE TAKE breathing for granted, it is rare that we would ever consider poor breathing habits as the source of our lack of energy, our nervous tension, our inability to concentrate, our bad heart, insomnia, lack of endurance, stomach problems or poor skin. Yet it is breathing—more than the food we eat, the amount of exercise we do—that affects how we think and feel. Breathing and the oxygen it provides affects every single cell in our body. Every one of our 100 trillion cells requires a continual supply of high-quality oxygen. It is this oxygen that feeds our brain, sparks our heart and calms our nerves.

We tend to think of breathing as just the mere inhalation and exhalation of air into and out of the body. Yet breathing is one of the greatest tools and resources influencing the vitality of our body and positively affecting our emotions. By breathing in specific ways we can set our busy mind to rest, change our mood, increase our prolongevity, reduce stress, wake up alert without three cups of coffee, concentrate better, improve our resistance to colds and respiratory infections, reduce our chance of heart disease and sleep a deeper, more thorough sleep.

From the moment we are born until the time we die, our breathing is one of the most important factors in keeping our body alive and well. Too many of us are poor breathers, cheating our body of the very oxygen that keeps it alive.

Each of us breathes in specific ways that are unlike anyone else's breathing patterns, which are as unique and individualistic as our fingerprints. Each emotion has a unique breathing pattern all its own. If we are tense or afraid, our breathing becomes quick and shallow. During relaxation and sleep our breathing becomes deep and regular, infusing the body with high-quality oxygen. The way we breathe affects how we think and feel, while the way we think and feel affects the way we breathe.

Breathing is one of the most complex, essential and controllable processes of the body. Primarily it is a medium of transportation, a process for oxygenating the body and removing carbon dioxide, the by-product of cellular activity. The entire functioning of our body is intimately connected with the process of breathing.

Both the heart and the blood, which oversee the maintenance of the body's internal environment, rely totally on the breath to supply them with oxygen and remove gaseous waste. Unlike other nutrients that feed the body such as vitamins, minerals and proteins, oxygen cannot be stored within the body and must continually be replenished. Every minute that we are alive we require steady and constant provisions of fresh oxygen. On the average we breathe about fifteen times a minute. What makes the respiration process unique in our body is that it functions both automatically and voluntarily. Unlike the flow of our blood or the beat of our heart, we are able to change the rate and pattern of our breath whenever we wish. The breathing process is also designed to operate completely on its own, without interference for the rest of our lives.

Through controlling and changing the way we breathe, we can better regulate the needs of our body. Because the breathing process is so intimately connected with our every thought and action, by mastering it we can continually monitor and improve our health, vitality and emotions. Through awareness of the way we breathe we can gain greater insight into the minute-by-minute workings of our body.

This book will teach you the right way to breathe for every aspect of your life, from sports and health to increased energy and relaxation. The exercises in this book require no special equipment or clothing. They can be performed anywhere and at any time. There are exercises to help you stay alert at the office, to improve your appearance and to induce sleep safely.

Each of the exercises is designed to perform a specific function. Though they may appear simple, the way in which the exercises introduce oxygen into the body is extremely important and can produce many beneficial results. Follow the directions carefully. Once you begin the programs you will notice a great many changes in the way you feel. As your breathing becomes deeper and fuller, you will find an overall increase in your level of well-being.

Initially you may find yourself becoming somewhat obsessive about your breathing. You will continually be checking it to see how you are breathing and in what ways you can improve your breathing. This will soon pass. Once you train yourself in proper breathing, it will rapidly become second nature. Eventually, as the body becomes accustomed to the increase in oxygen, you will find the body regulating its breathing pattern as needed.

Because most people do not know how to use their breathing, the exercises in this book are very specific and should be followed as written. If, after completing the entire book, you feel constrained by certain of the routines and you feel that you can improve upon them, feel free to modify the exercises so that they work comfortably for you. The important thing is to become aware of the importance of breathing and how it can always be used to improve your health and vitality.

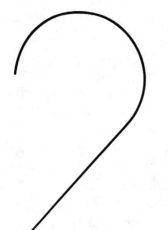

TOTAL BREATHING

THE FOUR MAIN TYPES of breathing are defined by the respiratory muscles used. They are *high breathing, mid breathing, low breathing,* and *total breathing.*

High breathing, unfortunately, is one of the most prevalent forms of breathing. Most of us are high breathers, especially if we have sedentary occupations. Whenever we sit or lean over our desk to work, the chest and stomach area tend to collapse in, thus preventing the full inflation of the entire lung area. A high breather characteristically breathes in a quick and shallow fashion in an attempt to provide the lungs with sufficient oxygen.

The old saying that doing something the wrong way takes more effort than doing it the right way is especially applicable in the case of high breathers. High breathing requires a great deal more effort to supply the body with enough oxygen than breathing properly and deeply. High breathing concentrates the inhalations in the upper chest area, which holds the smallest amount of air. This of course means poor oxygenation for the body. Breathing in this manner lifts only the upper ribs and not the most important muscle in the respiration process, the diaphragm. By breathing with just the upper chest, a great deal of stale air tends to accumulate in the rest of the lungs. Aside from inhibiting the intake of oxygen, the lungs may begin to atrophy by losing much of their important elasticity. With improper ventilation one greatly increases one's susceptibility to contagious diseases and upper respiratory complications.

Demonstrate for yourself the inadequacies of high breathing. Standing or sitting erect, first raise your shoulders and collarbone and then inhale. Another method is to sit at your desk and lean forward as if reading or writing. Now inhale. In both examples you will find that you can breathe only as far down as your upper breast. The breath seems suddenly to stop short while the rest of your lungs remain unfilled. You can clearly see and feel how limited a method of respiration high breathing is. Later, when you learn the method of total breathing, you might want to compare the differences in oxygen intake and lung expansion with high breathing. You will never return to insufficient breathing again.

Mid breathing is only a slight improvement over high breathing in terms of the amount of oxygen taken into the body. In addition to the top part of the lungs used in high breathing, mid breathing extends the breath down to the mid-section in the area of the ribs. To demonstrate mid breathing, lift the entire rib cage, then inhale. You will feel the breath reach farther down to the base of the rib section. Also notice that as you lifted the rib cage upward the stomach was slightly pulled in.

When the doctor tells you to "take a deep breath" and you breathe all the way to your stomach, you are practicing low breathing. Even though the lungs are employed far more extensively in low breathing than in any of the other forms of breathing, they are far from being completely filled with vital and necessary oxygen.

Total breathing is the most complete form of breathing. It fills the lungs to their maximum and uses every respiratory muscle. Total breathing employs all aspects of the previous three forms of breathing and then some. Not only are the chest and ribs lifted but also the intercostal muscles expand the ribs outward, providing a large space in which the lungs can be inflated to their maximum. To complete the fullness of this breath, the diaphragm enlarges further outward and pulls the lower ribs downward, which allows the very bottom part of the lungs, the largest and least used part of the lungs, to be filled completely with fresh air. As you can see, every possible cubic centimeter is used, along with a large percentage of chest, rib and stomach muscles.

Total breathing will form the basis for the majority of our breathing work because of its complete use of the respiratory muscles and the many benefits that are derived from the increased oxygen intake and carbon dioxide release. By using total breathing in our various breathing programs we will be providing our lungs with a substantial oxygen base, ridding the body of toxins and supplying increased amounts of oxygen to every cell in our body.

Practice the following instructions for the total breath until it becomes an automatic way of breathing. Throughout the book we will show you how to put this method of breathing to your best use. You will discover through the practice of this one exercise how much breathing can affect your health and well-being.

■ **TOTAL BREATH**

1. Inhale slowly through the nose, directly aiming the breath about two inches below the belly button. This will fill the *lower* part of the lungs with air. As you do this your stomach will begin to bulge out like a balloon. See Fig. 1.
2. As you continue the breath, fill the rest of the stomach area, then expand the rib section outward to the sides and fill the mid-section of the chest with air. See Fig. 2.
3. Finally, let the breath fill the uppermost part of the lungs by lifting up the chest area and letting it expand outward and to the side. The entire process should take about five seconds. See Fig. 3.

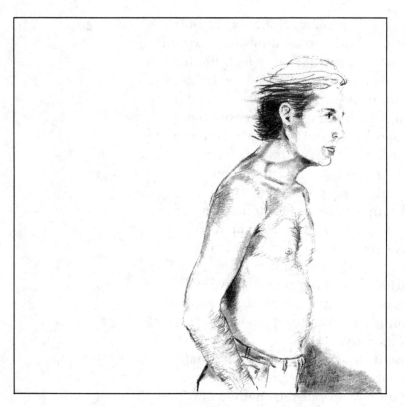

Fig. 1. Total Breath, Step 1.
Relax your stomach and allow it
to bulge out as you fill the lower
lungs with air.

4. Now hold the breath for five seconds. Eventually with practice you should hold the breath for ten seconds to give the lungs a good chance to use and absorb all the oxygen.

5. To exhale, follow the process used for inhalation. Begin by gently contracting the lower stomach first. This will push out the air in the lowest part of the lungs that will automatically carry with it the remaining air. As the lower lungs empty themselves of their air, the rib section will slowly deflate, followed by the upper chest. The exhalation should be done as slowly as the inhalation.

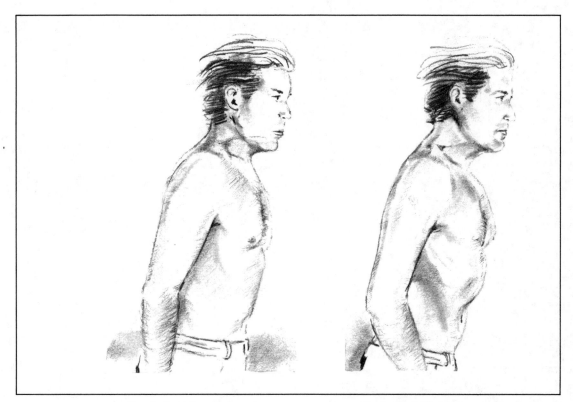

Fig. 2. Total Breath, Step 2.
Expand your ribs and let the
breath fill your mid-section.

Fig. 3. Total Breath, Step 3.
Continue the breath so that it
fills the upper chest and lungs.

6. Once you have completely finished the exhalation,
pause for a second or two before beginning the next
inhalation.

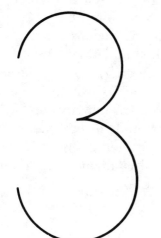

THE ENERGY PROGRAM

IN ESTABLISHING THE ENERGY base of the body we must provide a steady intake of fresh oxygen. Most of us employ our lungs at only one-third their potential capacity. They have to be re-educated into accepting and utilizing greater amounts of oxygen. Our regular habits of lazy respiration must be replaced by the most effective method of breathing possible, the *total breath.* In this way we can extract as much oxygen as our lungs will allow with each and every breath. This means, of course, added energy for every tissue and cell throughout the body. As we breathe with the total breath we will find ourselves being less tired, with a reserve of energy throughout the day. No longer will we feel as if we are on our last legs. With increased oxygen our bodies will be functioning better and more efficiently, like a finely tuned machine.

The exercises in the *energy program* are designed to supplement the total breath. They are to be used whenever fatigue begins to set in. Their purpose is quickly to restore declining oxygen levels throughout the body and brain which can seriously interfere with our performance. This infusion of high-quality oxygen will quickly restore our sense of vitality.

Whenever we feel ourselves becoming tired we immediately seek a sudden jolt of energy, such as a cup of coffee. These quick rushes of artificial stimulation have no real base on which to provide sustained energy over a period of time. Once they reach their peak, which is usually in about fifteen minutes, our bodies are then thrown into a valley of exhaustion. The *energizing breath* restimulates our energy base and provides steady waves of continued energy. Unlike coffee, it does so by bringing additional vitalizing oxygen into the body rather than chemical stimulation.

■ ENERGIZING BREATH

1. Sit comfortably in a chair and place your hands on your thighs.

2. Form your lips into an "O" and relax your tongue so that it does not block the passage of air. Now, quickly suck in through the mouth a total breath, filling first the lower part of the lungs, then the rib area and finally the upper chest. This should all be done in one quick, strong inhalation. Your breath should sound like a strong gust of wind. Your rib cage should be fully expanded and your posture fully erect.

3. Hold the breath for three seconds.

4. Exhale by forcefully blowing the breath out through the open mouth.

5. Repeat this sucking inhalation two more times.

6. On the last exhalation, gently blow the air out as if cooling a spoon of soup.

7. Repeat three times.

The energizing breath can be used at any time of the day when you feel the need for a quick pick-up. After three repetitions, the body will once again feel alert.

Fatigue most often occurs not because of the lack of energy but mainly because of the blockage of energy. Throughout the body are specific centers that supply us with continual levels of productive energy. As muscles contract with tension they tend to act like a steel net that interferes with the normal circulation of energy throughout the body. Negative or depressing thoughts also require enormous amounts of energy for their existence. Our thoughts and nervous actions can be as exhausting as a full day of hard exercise. We must always focus on efficient action and good feelings.

One of the most important factors in our energy production is the breath. As oxygen enters the body, it provides the fundamental fuel for the metabolic activities of the cells. If in any way we interfere with our oxygen intake, we inhibit the functioning of every system in the body. Thus we lack the incentive, drive and energy to get through the day-to-day. The energy supplied by the respiratory process affects the functioning of our brain, our stamina and our basic physical well-being. Through specific breathing exercises we can enhance both the quality and supply of our oxygen fuel.

Normally, we inhale just enough air to get by and keep ourselves functioning at a maintenance level. Even though we may feel fine, our body is not provided with sufficient fuel for it to function at peak capacity. In addition, normal breathing does little to remove the toxic build-up that occurs from the continual activity and wear and tear of the cells. This waste accumulates throughout the body unless it is regularly disposed of. If these toxins build up throughout the body they begin to interfere with our energy production. We soon feel sluggish and unmotivated.

The lungs function as one of the body's major excretory organs. With every exhalation, the breath removes carbon dioxide and other waste matter that has been converted into gaseous form. Unless our exhalations are full and deep, waste air containing the by-products of cellular activity remains at the base of the lungs. Over a time this stale air begins to accumulate, taking up important space in the lungs. This can severely inhibit our intake of fresh oxygen. As this condition develops, we find ourselves feeling stale. Our immediate response is to step outside for a breath of fresh air to refresh ourselves and to revive our declining energies.

Oftentimes our lack of energy is a result of the build-up of stale air in our lungs. The *full exhalation* helps clear this leftover air while at the same time providing the body with a fresh supply of energy-oxygen. It is the perfect exercise for alleviating that dull, tired feeling that often comes from being indoors all day.

■ FULL EXHALATION

1. Sitting, inhale the total breath. Toward the very end of the inhalation, straighten the back and pull up on the shoulders to insure a maximum intake of oxygen.
2. Hold for ten counts.
3. Open the mouth wide and exhale as much air as possible without straining. The exhalation should make a *haaa* sound. When you feel that you have completed the exhalation, close your mouth and inhale through the nose just a tiny sniff of air for two counts.
4. Again, open the mouth and exhale as fully as possible.
5. At the end of this exhalation, once more, close the mouth and inhale that sniff of air for two counts. Then, open the mouth and let out one last exhalation as fully as possible. To complete the exhalation, gently pull in on the lower abdomen to push out the remaining stale air. With each of the exhalations you should feel yourself breathing out from lower and lower portions of the lungs.
6. Repeat the entire exercise ten times. Each repetition should include the three full exhalations.

Most people think of energy in terms of a hyperkinetic frenzied state. However, living this way usually means thowing massive amounts of valuable energy into simple tasks or random thoughts, accomplishing little. What we are after is a calm, steady and ever-present supply of energy that is continually available. Rather than being all revved up with short-term spurts of power that leave wasted fuel and action in its wake, we seek a high-level energy state. With controlled breathing we can create a strong base of working energy that can recharge the body whenever necessary. The *vitalization breath* will slowly energize the body with fresh oxygen. The effects of this breath are gentle and long-lasting.

■ VITALIZATION BREATH

1. Sit comfortably in a chair and close your eyes.

2. Press your third finger into the middle of your forehead and close your right nostril with your right thumb. See Fig. 4.

3. Now, slowly inhale the total breath through the left nostril for ten counts.

4. With the fourth finger close the left nostril and hold the breath for ten counts.

5. To exhale, release only the thumb and slowly exhale through the right nostril for ten counts.

6. Pause for two counts.

7. Keeping the right nostril open, slowly inhale the total breath for ten counts.

8. Now, close the right nostril with the thumb and hold the breath for ten counts.

9. Exhale for ten counts by releasing the fourth finger only.

10. Pause for two counts. Continue the breath by alternating the nostrils until you have inhaled ten times through each side.

After finishing this exercise, you will feel calm waves of energy flowing through your entire body.

The *stimulant breath* is a powerful invigorator for the respiratory system and for the cells in the body. It aids the body in releasing locked clusters of energy. The first few times you practice the stimulant breath you may feel slightly dizzy or lightheaded. This is because you are releasing refined energy that your body is not accustomed to. After the exercise a wave of clean energy will sweep over the body, leaving you revitalized and alert.

■ STIMULANT BREATH

1. Standing straight, inhale the total breath deeply and slowly.

2. As you inhale, lightly tap your chest in various places with your fingertips. You should be making a "pitter

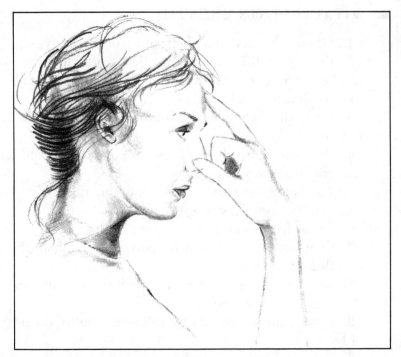

Fig. 4. Vitalization Breath, Step 2. Aim the breath toward the center of your forehead.

patter" sound as your hands dance across the chest. See Fig. 5.

3. When the lungs are filled, hold the breath for a count of fifteen. As you hold the breath, pat the chest with the palms of your hands. See Fig. 6.

4. Now exhale very slowly.

5. Repeat five times.

The *eyes-open breath* is good for a quick recharge of the body. It is especially useful as a break from work or studying.

■ EYES-OPEN BREATH

1. Sitting down, close your eyes and lean slightly forward in your chair with your hands resting on your knees.

2. Now, suddenly sit up straight and, as you do so, quickly sniff in the total breath. The force of the breath should push you back slightly in your chair. As you lean back, open your eyes as wide as they will go. Hold the eyes wide open and retain the breath for six counts.

3. Remain leaning back in your chair, make an "O" shape with your lips and blow out the breath as if you were sighing with relief. Now blink your eyes a few times.

4. Repeat the entire process three times.

Along with the neck, one of the main bottlenecks of our energy flow is the spine. If we sit at a desk all day or if we sleep on a soft mattress, the spine tends to become misaligned, which greatly interferes with the movement of important nerve messages throughout the body. The *stretch breath* quickly loosens up the spine while infusing the body with oxygen.

Fig. 5. Stimulant Breath, Step 2. Lightly tap your chest with your fingertips.

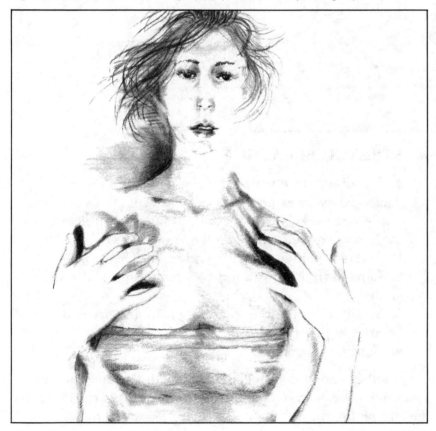

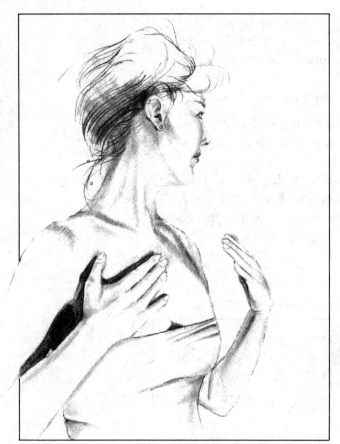

Fig. 6. Stimulant Breath, Step 3. Gently slap your chest with flat open hands.

■ STRETCH BREATH

1. Standing, place your hands on your hips and bend backward as far as possible. Let the weight of your head guide you backward. Notice the wonderful stretching and loosening you feel all along the spine. As you bend backward, open your mouth and exhale. See Fig. 7.
2. Remain in this position for as long as possible without strain.
3. Slowly return to the standing position. As you do so breathe in the total breath.
4. Repeat three times.

Another variation of the stretch breath that may prove easier for some who have difficulty in the backward stretch is the *stretch breath II.*

■ STRETCH BREATH II

1. Standing with your feet two feet apart, inhale the total breath and hold.

2. Place your hands on your upper thighs with your palms in, fingers pointing down.

3. Bend backward as far as possible and fully exhale. Use your hands for support. Let them slide down your thighs as you bend backward. Try to bend as far back as possible. Ideally your fingertips should come to rest on the insides of your knees. Hold for three counts.

4. As you slide back up, begin to inhale the total breath. Finish the inhalation once you are standing erect. Hold for ten counts.

5. Now repeat the exhalation of step three.

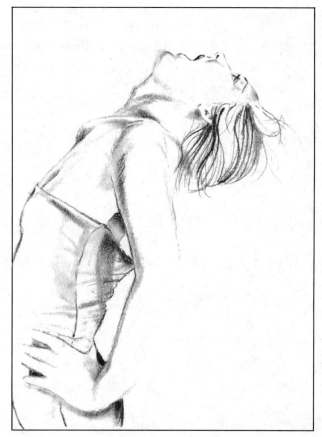

Fig. 7. Stretch Breath, Step 1. Bend backward as far as you can and exhale.

6. Repeat five times.

7. At the end of the exercise, inhale and exhale the total breath.

As you begin to explore the energy program, you will notice that the subtle shifts in your energy patterns will affect your mental states as well. A vital body can only produce dynamic thoughts and actions. As you refine the breath, thus supercharging the body, you will find yourself needing less and less stimulation by excess foods, coffee and drugs. The energy program should become a lifelong habit.

Because each person experiences energy in an individual way, we have provided a variety of breathing exercises all designed to stimulate the body's vitality. Some of the exercises may be exactly what you need, while others may be over- or understimulating. Experiment with each of the exercises over a period of weeks and in various situations. Eventually you will be able to discern the different ways each exercise affects your energy level. At that point you can choose the exercises which work best for you.

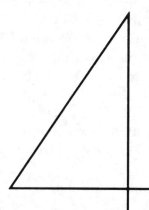

SPORTS PROGRAM

SURPRISINGLY, few athletes are aware of the important relationship between breath and performance. It is extremely rare that a coach will provide breathing exercises and techniques as part of an overall training program. Most people assume that their breathing will follow or at least keep up with their athletic performance. Even though the heart rate, circulation and the rate of respiration automatically increase with exertion, this natural response may not be enough to provide that extra push of strength when needed.

Probably more than any other factor, proper breathing is crucial to success in sports. During sports, oxygen serves as the body's major source of fuel. Our oxygen requirements increase at least tenfold during any physical exertion. This means that every cell in your body is in need of extra nutrients, more energy and increased metabolic exchange. The entire body is under pressure to keep all systems operating at maximum potential. Inadequate supplies of oxygen from improper breathing can seriously interfere with strength, endurance, flexibility and concentration. Training, skill and coordination can quickly be rendered useless if the body is not receiving substantial amounts of oxygen.

By following this sports breathing program you can affect the success of your athletic performance in two vitally important ways. First, you will be able to train your body to take in and utilize greater supplies of high-quality oxygen for increased endurance, stamina and strength. Second, you will learn to establish rhythmic breathing patterns which will provide the timing to which you will coordinate your every movement.

During sports, we have increased fuel requirements in order to supply the energy and meet the needs of physical stress. Every part of the body is being pushed to meet the requirements of physical exertion. With the body working at peak capacity, it is especially crucial that it be thoroughly oxygenated.

With this increase in physical activity, the body generates added amounts of carbon dioxide. Carbon dioxide is a waste product that, if not immediately disposed of through proper breathing, begins to build up in the bloodstream. This leaves less room for the incoming fresh oxygen that is so vitally needed. With more carbon dioxide and less oxygen in the body, fatigue quickly sets in. The presence of too much carbon dioxide can also lead to physical complications. As the toxins accumulate the athlete may find himself having problems with tendons, wrists, elbows, knees and ankles—the most important body parts for sports performance.

Coordination is one of the most important requirements for success in sports. During a play we are usually so caught up in where our hands should be, how hard to hit the ball, when to speed up and when to slow down that we are unable to unify our actions. Rhythmic breathing can set the basic pace with which we coordinate every movement for improved efficiency, impact and, ultimately, winning. Instead of worrying about ten things at once—where the opponent is standing, how fast to run or when to jump—all you do is breathe. The body and the game then take care of themselves. Each movement follows the next in graceful succession. By timing your movements with your breath you develop an integrated approach to sports. Concentration then becomes easy and focused. All of the distractions that usually arise during sports disappear with each breath.

■ RUNNING

Jogging is one of the better activities for encouraging full use of the respiratory system. With sustained running the heart works harder, pumping more blood throughout the body, and oxygen intake is thus increased. Since improved respiration is one of the natural effects of jogging, it is worth disciplining your breath to aid in this process. Through proper warm-up, breathing and various running breaths, you will be able to further your distance, increase your stamina and greatly enhance the cardiovascular effects of running. Many people who have been running for years, including marathon runners, completely ignore the importance of proper breathing for successful and beneficial running. Little do they realize the various stages that the breath goes through from warm-up to cool-down. Few runners realize that breathing can improve their running far more than the best running shoes. Most of them let their breath follow its own separate course—too often and too quickly becoming "out of breath" as a result. There are specific breathing techniques that are used for warm-up, for increasing endurance, for long-distance running and for reviving waning energy.

Probably the simplest and most effective breathing technique to use during running is the total breath, which will provide you with a smooth and constant supply of oxygen. By correcting your breathing you will avoid such common runners' problems as side stitch, shortness of breath and fatigue. The total breath should be considered your basic running breath.

Inhalation for the total breath takes place in three parts. First, the stomach is pushed outward to accommodate as much air as possible in the lower part of the lungs. Then the ribs are lifted up and to the sides to fill the middle part of the lungs. Finally the upper chest area is lifted and filled. These three steps should be performed as one smooth single inhalation. The exhalation is just the reverse of the inhalation. Begin by pulling in the lower stomach, which forces out the bulk of the air. Once you start the exhalation mechanism, the ribs and the upper chest will naturally follow, emptying themselves of their air. While it is preferable to breathe through the nose, the total breath can be done through the mouth while running.

■ TOTAL BREATH FOR RUNNING

1. To inhale, push the stomach out and let the air rush in to fill the lower lungs. Let the breath progressively fill the rib-cage area and finally the upper chest. Be sure to expand your rib cage out as far as possible to allow in a good supply of air.

2. To exhale, slightly contract the stomach and then let the air release itself progressively from the mid area and then the chest areas.

3. Continue breathing in this fashion as you run.

To prevent cramping as well as to establish a steady rhythm to sustain you during the run, each inhalation and exhalation should be done slowly to the count of ten. Keeping the count mentally focuses the attention on a steady rhythm and keeps your mind off feelings of fatigue or anxiety. This leaves the body free to fall naturally into its best running form unencumbered by tiring or distracting thoughts. No matter whether you choose to run quickly or leisurely, you should maintain the same steady number of counts for each inhalation and exhalation. As a demonstration to yourself of the importance and benefits of this breathing method, compare your regular running breath with the total breath for running. The comparison can be done at home in a few minutes. Run in place for a few minutes and breathe as you usually do while running. Most likely the breath will be concentrated mainly in the chest area. Then rest for a few minutes until you feel refreshed. Again, run in place but use the total breath. You will notice that when you breathe correctly you need fewer breaths, your endurance is vastly improved and running becomes effortless. After this demonstration you will realize it makes absolutely no sense to breathe incorrectly during the run. The investment of just a few minutes to learn the total breath thoroughly will change the way you run.

Usually after a period of running the body tends to bend over slightly from fatigue, thus restricting the rise and fall of the chest and inhibiting the full flow of oxygen into the lungs. Needless to say, this only increases fatigue. At this point you want to revive the muscle tone of the chest as well as pump more air into and out of the body. The *two-part breath* will quickly remove the increasing build-up of carbon dioxide as well as return the body to proper breathing. While running, remember to use your breath as a guiding instrument. With proper use, the breath will provide you with all the pacing and energy you will need. If during the run you feel in need of more air, switch over to the two-part breath, concentrate on full exhalations and the inhalations will come naturally.

■ TWO-PART BREATH

1. When fatigue sets in, it is crucial to get as much carbon dioxide out of the body as possible. This can be done by increasing your exhalations. As you run, breathe out through the mouth in a huff as if you were blowing out a candle.

2. Breathe in through the nose, filling the lungs with the total breath.

3. Pull up the chest, straightening the neck and the head, and sniff in an extra bit of air for the upper lungs. This will reinstate the proper posture of the body and add extra oxygen to the bloodstream. Even though the inhalation is in two parts, it should be performed as one smooth movement, with just the slightest pause between the first inhalation and the upper lung sniff.

In a marathon your body is operating at peak capacity. All systems are pushed beyond normal requirements. The critical factors for long-distance running are endurance and strength, both of which depend on the way you breathe. Through controlled breathing you can feed your body supercharged oxygen, the important fuel which will provide the reserve energy when you are about to tire. Even though other factors play a large role in your performance such as training, diet, the amount of sleep you got and your desire to win, correct breathing could make the critical difference as to *when* you cross the finish line.

During running, especially long-distance running, it is important not to let yourself get into the habit of panting with an open mouth for breath. This happens when your oxygen requirement is extremely high. Panting is the body's attempt to get as much oxygen into the body as quickly as possible because your regular breathing has not been doing the job. If you feel you absolutely must breathe through the mouth, then make sure that it is a slow and full inhalation rather than a shallow pant.

One veteran runner uses the breath as a diversionary tactic during major marathons. Whenever he is running next to a competitor he begins to pant rapidly as if he were severely out of breath. This trick gives the competitor a false sense of confidence while subverting his breathing pattern. If the competitor is not monitoring his own breath, he may suddenly find himself out of breath with no explanation.

One of the most annoying yet common problems during long runs is the appearance of a seemingly unquenchable thirst. Being thirsty while running can make the finish line seem a million miles away. The *thirst breath* given on page 165 will quickly relieve the thirst while cooling the body and make breathing easier.

Often runners experience a pain in their ribs while running. Rather than stopping because of this pain it is best to run through it. Increase the depth of your inhalations and most importantly the exhalations. You will find if you thoroughly force all the air out of your lungs during the exhalation, the pain will quickly subside. It may return on subsequent occasions, but each time it will last for shorter and shorter durations. Eventually by increasing your lung capacity the pain will disappear. That sticking in the ribs tends to cause you to inhibit your breathing. You then find yourself breathing from the upper chest in order to avoid pain. This only prolongs the condition. Deep breathing below the pain is exactly what you need. Above all, do not stop running when the pain appears. You may wish to slow down a bit, but keep your breathing working till the pain subsides.

■ WARM-UP

Probably more important than the effort you put into running that daily mile is the effort you put into the warm-up before you start to run. Too often time-conscious people forego the warm-up session because of supposed lack of time. They don't realize that warming up is an important form of exercise that can be done in as little as three minutes. By preparing the body for exercise you increase your potential for maximum performance and greatly eliminate the possibility of injury. In the warm-up your breathing increases that important supply of oxygen to the muscles as they begin to stretch themselves out and prepare themselves for physical activity. The focus of any warm-up is to gear up the respiratory system, eliminate as much carbon dioxide as possible and to loosen up the muscles. The following warm-up breaths are applicable to any sport and should be performed before any physical activity.

■ HANDCLASP

This exercise primes the body with extra oxygen while at the same time loosening up the spine and upper torso.

1. Standing, interlock the fingers of both hands, raise your arms above the head and turn them inside out (palms up).
2. Inhale the total breath. Then, lift the hands and stretch the body upward as far as they will go and inhale a second time to fill the top of the lungs.
3. Now, bend sideways to the right as far as you can and let the breath out in a long sniff. See Fig. 8.

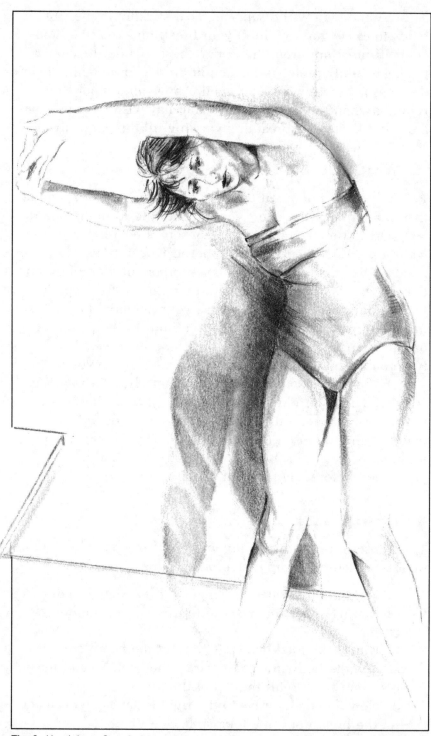

Fig. 8. Handclasp, Step 3. As you exhale, let the body stretch as far to the right as possible.

4. Straighten back up, inhale, lift the hands and inhale a second time.

5. Bend sideways to the left as far as you can and let the breath out in a sniff.

6. Straighten up, inhale, lift the hands and inhale a second time.

7. Repeat ten times each side.

■ KICKING AND BREATHING

The kicks give you the opportunity to coordinate movement and breath. Kicking to the side stretches out the entire leg, preventing the muscles from bunching up during the run.

1. Stand with hands on hips with legs spread eighteen inches apart.

2. Using the right leg as support, lift the left leg straight out and away from the body. Fully exhale as you lift the leg and inhale as the leg returns. Repeat ten times.

3. Now, using the left leg as support, lift the right leg straight out and away from the body. Fully exhale as you lift the leg and inhale as the leg returns. Repeat ten times with each leg.

■ BENDING BREATH

1. Stand with hands on hips, legs about eighteen inches apart.

2. Inhale the total breath.

3. Without bending the knees, bend forward from the waist, keeping your trunk straight. As you bend forward, exhale through the mouth with a single quick breath.

4. As you come back up, sniff in a lung full of air.

5. Pause momentarily and again bend forward and exhale.

6. Continue the exercise for fifteen counts.

■ DANGLE BREATH

The dangle breath is one of the most complete forms of stretching. It loosens the spine, especially the lower back, which can cause any number of problems during athletics. It also provides a fresh supply of blood and oxygen to the brain, getting rid of any feelings of fatigue or cloudy thinking. During step three while you dangle you may swing your arms from side to side or back and forth between your legs if you wish.

1. Standing with your feet about eighteen inches apart, inhale the total breath.
2. From the waist upward, let the body fall toward the floor and just dangle. As the body drops downward, expel all the breath in one large exhalation through the open mouth.
3. As you let your head just hang, feel the stretch going up the back of your legs, loosening up your lower back and your spine, stretching out vertebra by vertebra. Hang for ten counts.
4. Begin your inhalation as you come up. It should be completed by the time you are standing erect.
5. Repeat ten times.

Another variation of the dangle that produces different effects in terms of oxygen supply is the *sniffing breath*.

■ SNIFFING BREATH

The sniffing breath gives you the same muscular stretch and toning as the dangle breath. The main difference lies in the method of inhalation that conditions the lungs and prepares them for the ensuing stress.

1. Standing with your feet about eighteen inches apart, inhale the total breath.
2. Bend from the waist, letting the torso fall toward the floor and just hang. As the body drops downward, expel all the breath in one large exhalation through the open mouth.

3. Let your body hang for ten counts.

4. Bring the body up vertebra by vertebra. Each time you raise the body a notch, inhale a sniff of air. When you are standing straight, lift your arms above your head to finish the inhalation.

5. Keep your arms up and hold the breath for ten counts.

6. Drop your arms to your side and let the air rush out of your mouth.

7. Inhale once again through your nose the total breath.

8. Drop your upper body and exhale. Continue the exercise.

9. Repeat ten times.

■ HISSING BREATH

The *hissing breath* is important to clear out fully the remnants of stale air in the lungs. This decreases the possibility of becoming short of breath or incurring fatigue. By cleaning out the lungs, you are also making more room for greater quantities of oxygen, which promotes greater stamina and better performance during the run.

1. Inhale the total breath.

2. Tilt your head back so that your chin is pointing up in the air.

3. Open your lips and force the exhalation out between closed teeth, making a hissing sound.

4. Bring the head back down and inhale.

5. Tilt the head back and repeat exhalation.

6. Repeat ten times.

It is crucial to ease the body out of its athletic condition and back to normalcy after physical exertion. This means that all the systems, from cardiovascular and muscular to respiratory and circulatory, must pass through a transition phase so that none of them goes into shock. For example, if you immediately stop moving after running, the body is left with a pounding heart and all the systems functioning at peak capacity. By gradually winding down you slip back into normal operations without stressing the body.

After any sport in which you have exerted yourself, you will naturally be tired and thirsty. At this point the worst possible thing you could do is to lie down and gulp a gallon of ice water, neither of which the body is prepared for. There is a method of breathing that will relieve thirst and also return the breathing rate to normal. After the run, keep walking; do not stop. And as you are walking perform the thirst breath to help satisfy your craving for fluids.

■ THIRST BREATH

1. Pull the tongue back and place it against the upper palate.
2. Form your lips into a wide grin and suck in the air through the mouth. See Fig. 9.
3. Close the mouth.
4. Exhale through the nose.
5. Swallow.
6. Repeat until the thirst disappears.

You may wish to alternate the thirst breath with the total breath. During long runs if thirst suddenly overcomes you and all you can think about is having a large glass of water, try the thirst breath a few times and the urge will quickly disappear.

All sports require enhanced breathing and additional oxygenation. We must be able to inflate our lungs to their maximum in order to secure as much oxygen as possible, which will remove much of the fatigue-producing toxic wastes. The *lung enhancement breath* provides a good build-up program for the lungs.

■ LUNG ENHANCEMENT BREATH

1. Inhale a total breath.
2. Hold.
3. With closed fists pound the upper chest area, all down the chest, including the ribs and the upper abdomen. Pound for as long as you can comfortably hold the breath.

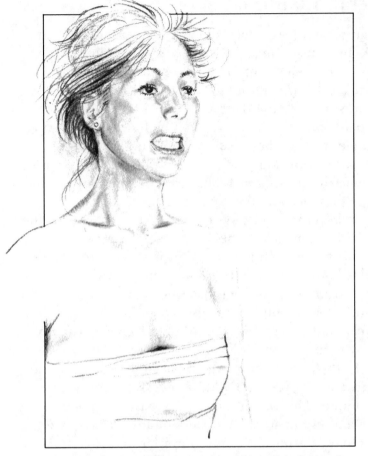

Fig. 9. Thirst Breath, Step 2. As you quickly suck in the breath through closed teeth, you will feel a cooling sensation at the back of your throat.

4. Stop pounding and exhale slowly through the nose.
5. Inhale a total breath, hold for five seconds and exhale.
6. Inhale the total breath and repeat entire process again.
7. Repeat three times.

This breath stimulates and opens up locked passageways for air. It should be periodically incorporated either into your warm-up or cooling-off period as a method of improving lung capacity and muscle tone. After each exhalation your chest will be tingling and your breathing will be much easier and much deeper.

■ MENTAL TRAINING

Increasingly, major-league athletes employ various mental techniques in order to improve their playing ability. These range from self-hypnosis and mental visualization to meditation. We are beginning to realize that mental preparation is just as important as physical training for any game we play. Part of this preparation includes just relaxing into the game itself without worrying about winning the game or scoring well. Many athletes find that once they relax into the game the playing just takes care of itself, and in some strange way they become the game itself.

The whole purpose of physical training is to prepare the body for all the demands of the sport. In this way we eliminate various random factors of surprise from the game. Our muscles know how to spring into action, our bodies know how to run, turn and stop. Coaches have always used team meetings or planning sessions to develop game plans with the team and to "psych" them into action. We can do the same by sitting down, relaxing and mentally previewing the game. In this way we can watch our moves, imagine how our opponent would respond and, if necessary, correct any faulty technique. This method helps increase our playing confidence and eliminates the anxiety of any surprise we might encounter during the game. In order to derive full benefit from these mental previews we must first relax ourselves into a quiet, receptive state.

■ SPORTS PREVIEW

1. Sit or lie down, close your eyes and slowly inhale the total breath for ten counts. Focus your attention to the center of your forehead.
2. Hold for five counts.
3. Exhale for ten.
4. Repeat three more times.
5. Now, with your eyes still closed, picture yourself in your particular sport.

Notice the clothes you are wearing, as well as the way your competitor is dressed. Mentally picture the day, the field.

Now start the game (or the run), watching yourself play as you usually would. Be an objective observer, like a coach. If you see mistakes in form or technique, stop the mental film and tell the player (yourself) how to improve each play. Also be aware of your feeling during the game. Are you concerned about winning, do your muscles hurt, are you fatigued or out of breath? Again, talk to the player and tell him to relax, that he is in good shape. Give him professional tips on how he can improve his serve or how to hold his arms while running. Now remember, you are acting as a professional coach. Once all the suggestions have been made, mentally play the game again. This time it will be perfectly played, all errors corrected. Notice your form, how you handle the ball in tight situations and how quickly and effortlessly you are moving as you run. Also watch your opponent, study his form, read his mind about how he plans to win. Learn from him if you can or at least understand his techniques. During this preview your breathing may slow down quite a bit. Once you have made all the necessary corrections in your game, inhale a good total breath three times and open your eyes. Now forget about the process you have just gone through. You will see the results in your next game. Know that you have just finished an intensive coaching session with the best coach in the world.

The purpose of the sports preview is to familiarize yourself with your own abilities as an athlete. It gives you an opportunity to study your moves and to correct them. Importantly, the sports preview allows you to relax with yourself and the competition. By having already viewed the field and the other players you will not feel that gripping anxiety that inhibits your body as you tell yourself you have to win. In this way you coach your body as well as rid yourself of the fear that often causes athletes to fail.

Another very effective method of mentally preparing for competition is to give the body positive suggestions while in a relaxed state. These then become part of the subconscious and will help you to run faster, swim farther and maintain a high-energy level throughout the game. *Sports self-suggestion* can be used to direct the body to perform to your best expectations.

■ SPORTS SELF-SUGGESTION

1. Sit or lie down, close your eyes and slowly inhale the total breath for ten counts. Focus your attention to the center of your forehead.

2. Hold for ten counts.

3. Exhale for ten.

4. Repeat three more times.

5. Now, with your eyes still closed, feel the relaxation sweeping over your body, becoming more and more pleasant. You will feel as if you are gently floating deeper and deeper. This is the perfect state of concentration for making self-suggestions. The suggestion should be a simple sentence. Depending on your particular need, the suggestions might be "My body grows stronger every day." "I can swim eighty laps without tiring." "My backhand is now completely successful." "I can place the ball anywhere on the court." Make the suggestion only once while holding the breath. Say it very firmly and clearly.

6. You may sit quietly for as long as it is comfortable. Keep your mind completely free from other thoughts. Give the suggestion a chance to sink in. Then, breathe regularly.

7. When you are ready, open your eyes.

Sports self-suggestion can be done whenever you feel there is a particular area of your performance that you are not completely satisfied with. Next time you play or work out you will begin to notice the changes in your performance. They will occur automatically and unexpectedly. Suddenly you will find yourself running that extra mile and in shorter time.

■ WALKING AND HIKING

Walking and hiking are excellent exercises for the entire body, providing thorough stimulation to the circulation. Both require correct breathing as an aid to stamina and endurance, especially when you are covering miles of ground. As with running, the total breath is probably your best all-around breath to insure proper oxygenation of the body. Your breathing rate should be comfortable and leisurely, never too quick or too slow. A good measure of proper walking breathing is that your rate of breathing should never interfere with your ability to carry on a conversation. For walking and hiking an easy natural rhythm of movement and posture is crucial. The head should be floating nicely on the neck, not held with rigidity or cramped. The spine should be naturally erect but not to the point of strain. This will help you breathe in an unrestrained manner. For relaxation as you walk, pretend that you are watching a movie, that the scenery around you changes as the film unrolls. In many ways walking and hiking are quite therapeutic in that they give you the opportunity to think and relax as you give your body a chance to unwind.

■ WEIGHT LIFTING

Effective weight lifting is extremely dependent on a high oxygen supply for good results. Without proper breathing the development of muscle mass takes much longer, often at the expense of other parts of the body. To lift the weight you borrow fuel from other vital functions of the body. Thorough respiration in weight lifting helps oxygenate the body, pumping added fuel into the muscles so that they do not tire as quickly. Thus you can lift much longer, which naturally leads to better conditioning, greater muscle mass and improved strength. Most health clubs are now equipped with the various types of weight-lifting machines. They are calibrated to work specific muscles throughout the body. Whether you use these machines or regular weights, the breathing remains the same.

■ BREATHING FOR WEIGHT LIFTING: POWER BREATH

1. Form your mouth like an "O" and in three strong sniffs suck in a lungful of air.
2. As you press or lift, exhale forcefully through a slightly

opened mouth, with the lips formed as if you were going to whistle. The breath should come out like a gust of wind. Let the exhalation power the lift. This will prevent fatigue, reduce the strain and oxygenate the body, helping to build muscles.

■ TENNIS

In tennis, power and concentration can mean a successful backhand and forehand. Proper breathing should be used throughout the game to insure correct form and prevent fatigue. Many times during athletics, players are so concerned with winning that they retain their breath instead of fully exhaling. For any shot you should inhale the total breath as the arm moves backward in preparation for the swing. Do not fill the lungs so completely that the body becomes stiff because of an inflated rib cage. A normal breath will do. Smoothly exhale as you swing. This will enable you to focus your body and mind on the shot. As soon as you hit the ball, finish the exhalation in a single huff through an open mouth. This will give your hit more power and will force you to concentrate on the hit itself. Then close the mouth, inhale and prepare for the next shot. If your lung capacity is sufficiently developed and your game of tennis is fast enough, you should be able to time your breathing pattern with your swings.

Much work has been done with applied relaxation and visualization techniques in tennis. The breathing exercises of *sports preview* and *sports self-suggestion* are perfect for helping you improve your game from a mental standpoint.

■ SWIMMING

Improper breathing is the most common shortcoming of swimmers. We already know how important breathing is to provide increased endurance and fatigue-free muscles, both of which are crucial to swimming. Because swimming is a water sport, buoyancy is important in stopping fatigue and helping us glide through the water. Like an inner tube or life vest, our bodies can support a good amount of weight in the water when filled with air. Proper breathing can help the body float while we swim. This eliminates a great deal of dead weight that the arms and legs would ordinarily have to propel through the water. Because we have only a brief few seconds in which to take in a maximum amount of air, it helps if we have exercised and aerated our lungs and our rib cage before we swim. The lung-enhancement breath in this chapter is excellent in creating greater lung potential for swimming.

In swimming, the integration and coordination of various movements is extremely important for efficient swimming. The easiest way to make swimming a singular action is to coordinate all movements through the breathing.

Actually, breathing during swimming is a very natural and logical movement. As one arm begins to come out of the water and reach forward, that shoulder naturally rises. At this time, the head merely has to turn and lift slightly to come in contact with air in order to breathe and then submerge.

■ SWIMMING BREATH

1. As the right arm comes out of the water and begins to sweep the body forward it pulls the body to the right side.

2. Next, as the left shoulder rises out of the water, turn the nose and mouth to the left side, lift the head just slightly out of the water, open the mouth and breathe in as much air as possible.

3. As the left arm begins to catch the water, turn the forehead slightly, submerging it in the water.

4. As the left arm strokes, exhale through the nostrils. (Many beginners have difficulty exhaling under water, so it is best to practice nasal exhalation in shallow water before attempting to swim.)

5. As the right arm prepares to come out of the water again, turn the head to the right, lift the nose and mouth out of the water, breathe deeply and return the head to the water.

6. Complete the stroke with the right arm.

7. Exhale.

Backstroke breathing should be accomplished with as little head motion as possible. This keeps the balance of the swimmer and encourages speed. Breathing while doing the backstroke is a matter of alternating the inhalations and the exhalations as each arm comes out of the water. Breathe out as the first arm leaves the water and inhale as the second arm leaves the water. Continue this rhythm.

As with every other style of swimming, the breathing of the breast stroke is coordinated with the movement of the arms. As you begin the stroke with the hands coming forward and sweeping out to the sides, the head is lifted and the breath is taken in through the mouth. The arms then continue the stroke, and as they come together again for another thrust the head is lifted and the air is exhaled.

The butterfly also uses just the movement of the head for breathing without upsetting the movement of the body. Inhalation is always coupled with the forward movement of the arms. Breathing comes early in this stroke. Some coaches feel that it is not necessary to breathe regularly during the butterfly and that breaths should only be taken as needed. But breathing helps the body attain maximum speed with minimum effort, so you should work on coordinating it with your strokes.

■ LIFESAVING

If for some reason you should become stranded while swimming and too tired actually to swim, your breathing can keep you afloat.

■ BUOY BREATH

1. By inhaling a total breath you will supply the body with enough air to keep it afloat. Hold the breath and float as comfortably in the water as possible. To do so, keep your face in the water, look down and bend at the waist with your legs dangling downward. Your arms will also dangle downward. Float in this relaxed position until you feel you need a breath. To propel yourself to the surface, push yourself up and out of the water with your arms, while at the same time kicking your legs in a scissorslike motion.

2. Do not jump out of the water; merely raise yourself up far enough to get a lungful of fresh air. Return to your comfortable floating position.

The scissors kick can also be used to propel yourself slowly to the shore.

■ DIVING

Underwater diving is made possible through the creation of an artificial source of air. Respiration is the *key* factor that limits or encourages underwater diving. The diver using any underwater breathing apparatus should breathe deeply and slowly. This allows the oxygen to flow steadily into the body without sudden interruptions. By breathing this way the diver avoids complications that develop from an unsteady flow of air.

If the diver is performing tasks under water and finds himself running out of breath, it is urgent that he stop the work immediately until he regains control of his breath. In times of panic a diver may unconsciously begin to hyperventilate, and this can produce dizziness, nausea and possibly drowning. If at any time during the dive you feel slightly uncomfortable or that you are losing control, immediately take notice of your breathing. Consciously begin to take long slow breaths with full exhalations. This will normalize the high oxygen content that has occurred from hyperventilation. Divers may also forget to exhale fully after each breath. This can also produce dizziness and unconsciousness because of an elevated level of carbon dioxide in the system. Deep, steady breaths with full exhalations will remedy any faintness that might occur. Because of the possibility of passing out and drowning from too much oxygen or carbon dioxide in the bloodstream, the importance of correct breathing during scuba diving cannot be stressed enough.

It almost goes without saying that your oxygen supplies should be purchased from an experienced and reputable dealer. The mixture of air must be perfect. A ration of oxygen that is too concentrated or too weak can lead to oxygen poisoning. Oxygen poisoning often creeps upon you before you even have the opportunity to realize what is wrong. The symptoms are dizziness, nausea and blacking out.

Diving, along with all other sports, relies on increased lung capacities for stamina and endurance. But breathing is especially important in diving because of the dependence on tanked air; the body must utilize the limited supply of oxygen as effectively as possible. Developing good lung expansion and warm-up breathing exercises will greatly increase your ability as a diver. Many divers in their early training learn how to expand their lungs and hold the breath as long as possible. In this way the body becomes more adept in its use of oxygen under water. The lung enhancement breath given on page 32 in this chapter is extremely useful for expanding the lungs' breathing potential. It is good practice for all divers to increase the length of time for which they can hold their breath.

■ BREATH HOLDING I

1. Exhale completely by contracting the stomach, bringing it as far back toward the spine as possible.
2. Fully inhale the total breath. Close your eyes and begin counting to twenty. As you continue to count, raise your arms up over your head. This stretches the breath out so that it covers as much lung area as possible.
3. When you reach the count of twenty, slowly exhale through the nose as you lower your arms.
4. Repeat this exercise two more times. With each repetition, try to hold your breath for an additional five counts.

■ BREATH HOLDING II

This exercise is especially well suited to expanding the rib cage, thus increasing the room for lung expansion.

1. Inhale the total breath. Hold for twenty counts.
2. As you retain the breath, place your hands on your hips and pull your elbows back toward the spine as far as they will go. This movement will help increase chest expansion. See Fig. 10.
3. Repeat three times. With each repetition, try to hold the breath for an additional five counts.

In the beginning you may find it difficult to hold your breath for any amount of time. This, of course, is due to the lungs' lack of elasticity. During the breath-holding exercises don't concentrate on how long you have been holding your breath or how hard it is. Instead, direct your attention elsewhere. There are several techniques to redirect your concentration. Choose the one that is best suited for you. While you are holding your breath, look straight ahead with the eyes fixed exactly on some object. Use the object only as a focal point; do not study its details. (You could even look only at the tip of your nose.) While you are holding your breath, try to remain as physically and mentally relaxed as possible. Mental and muscular tension makes the process much more difficult. When you feel you *must* exhale, quickly check the upper chest area and shoulder for tension before you do so. You may find the area tensed up, and by just relaxing you may be able to hold your breath much longer.

Breath holding should only be practiced on land as a method of stretching and exercising your lungs. The most important rule to know in diving is, *never hold your breath underwater.* While using underwater breathing apparatus make sure you breathe regularly. Because of the pressure changes that occur during the dive and their effect on the air in the lungs, you stand a very good chance of bursting your lungs if you hold your breath. Once such a rupture occurs, air begins to bubble into the bloodstream, which can easily cause death. Some divers in an attempt to stretch their air

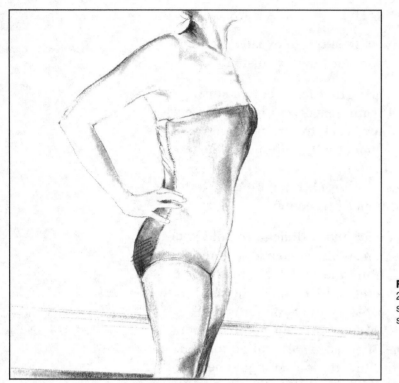

Fig. 10. Breath Holding II, Step 2. Pulling the elbows back will stretch your upper chest and spine.

supply often hold their breaths longer than they should. This is a fallacious practice that causes a build-up of carbon dioxide in the lungs which forces you to breathe more. Holding the breath can also cause the air to creep into spaces under the skin.

Probably the second most important rule in diving is that it should never be done alone. The reason for this rule is simple: There are just too many dangers. Having a buddy nearby to help you can really save your life. One of the greatest lifesaving functions a buddy can perform is helping you breathe if your air supply should fail. *Buddy breathing*, when diving partners share a single air tank, can help a stranded diver in a time of emergency.

■ BUDDY BREATHING

1. As soon as you discover that your air systems are in trouble, motion to your buddy. Symbolically slice your

throat with your finger to let him know that your air supply has been cut off. Then take your mouthpiece out of your mouth to show him that you are indeed in trouble. Point from your mouthpiece to his mouthpiece.

2. Get together with your buddy. Each of you should place your left hand on each other's shoulder for support so that you don't drift away.

3. After your buddy inhales he will hand you his mouthpiece. Once it is in your mouth, exhale the breath you were holding. Then inhale a fresh breath, exhale and inhale. Return the mouthpiece to your buddy.

4. To prevent wasting time and precious air between passes of the mouthpiece, it is a good idea to hold onto the mouthpiece together with your buddy.

5. Continue this shared breathing as you both begin your ascent.

Diving can also be performed with a snorkel tube and diver's mask. You breathe through the snorkeling tube while the mask lets you survey the underwater scene without submerging yourself in water. If you wish to dive below the water to take a closer look, breathe in a full inhalation through the tube, hold your breath and dive downward. You can stay under as long as you can hold your air. As you surface, exhale through the tube to blow out the accumulated water and begin breathing through the snorkel as before.

5

STOP-SMOKING PROGRAM

PRIMARILY, SMOKING is a fantasy. There is no such thing as one "has to have" a cigarette to relax, gain confidence, concentrate or look interesting. These are all false concepts that have entered the popular imagination through the images of advertising. Cigarette ads dating back to the 1930s and 1940s showed brave fighting men smoking on their way into battle, and even doctors wholeheartedly recommending menthol cigarettes for the health of their patients. The various mental associations that make one smoke are only myths dreamed up by Madison Avenue. It seems that if they can get people to accept a behavior as nonsensical as smoking as being enjoyable, they could just as easily induce them into chewing rocks for dessert.

Most smokers are instantly on the defensive whenever the issue is raised because in all sincerity they would much rather not be smoking. They would prefer to relax, gain confidence and look interesting in some other way. On top of which they would probably rather use all the money they spend every day on cigarettes to have a bottle of champagne once a week instead. But despite all the other less expensive and more healthful pleasures available in life, people still continue to smoke for any number of pointless reasons.

Few people stop to consider the fact that smoking is dependent on the breath for its effects. One does not enjoy the psychological and physiological lifts from a cigarette if it is put in your ear, between your toes or just held in your mouth. It has to be involved with your respiratory system in some way.

■ SMOKING WORKS BECAUSE IT MAKES YOU BREATHE

Primarily people smoke because they wish to relieve anxiety that is often accompanied by a tightness in the chest; they want a break from work or desire a "lift." All of these sensations are achieved by smoking because when you light the cigarette you *inhale,* usually quite deeply. And when you *exhale,* you breathe out the smoke quite smoothly and steadily. Both are like a sigh of relief. This means that through smoking you are taking in additional oxygen as well as breathing out excess carbon dioxide. Smoking cleverly gets people to use their own breathing for relaxation. Unfortunately it's a rather damaging way to breathe.

Smoking and the craving to smoke form one of those vicious circles that perpetuate themselves. Smoking and the need for smoking tend to reinforce each other continually. During any form of anxiety, breathing tends to become shallow and restricted to the upper chest area. This is a sign that the body is not being properly oxygenated and that carbon dioxide is not adequately being removed. At this point the lungs are hardly being used. As this shallow breathing continues, we become increasingly tense. The muscles in our neck and back become as hard as steel. Our stomach becomes a mass of burning cement. Our clarity of thought is undermined by lack of oxygen in the brain, by physical discomfort and by the anxiety of the situation itself. So instead of taking a few deep breaths which would alleviate the tension, we reach for a cigarette.

The cigarette makes us inhale deeply, which temporarily forces open the chest. With each inhalation of smoke we lift our rib cage, activate the diaphragm and stretch out the lungs. Following the exhalation of this first touch of cigarette smoke, we usually take a deep sigh of relief. This is when we feel that warm wave of relaxation washing over us. We use the cigarette as a way to stretch and breathe deeply. However, this feeling of relaxation is only temporary because each cigarette we smoke continues to restrict further our natural breathing. From the very first cigarette ever smoked the breathing becomes increasingly shallow until in the end it is reduced to mere panting. Our breath becomes restricted to the very top of the lungs. Our body becomes conditioned to breathing normally *only* with a cigarette. Thus the breathing/smoking cycle becomes established. What we have to learn is how to recognize and satisfy this need without reaching for a cigarette. Part of the reason that cigarettes help relieve tension is because we believe that *only* a cigarette will help us relax. We *must* realize that it is really *breathing* and not the cigarette that alleviates tension.

A great deal of smoking goes on in offices. Aside from the obviously tense atmosphere that often accompanies business, much of our time at work is spent hunched over a desk in a poorly ventilated environment. Notice that when you sit down to read or write at a desk your body tends to fold forward just about in the middle of the chest. In this position your breathing is focused on the top part of the lungs only. After a period of time the body has had it with insufficient oxygen and lack of movement and says "do something." We then reach for a cigarette in an effort to increase our intake of oxygen.

Cigarette smoke is a terribly complicated combination of poisonous gases and chemicals. It's actually quite amazing that after one cigarette we just don't keel over and drop dead. In the case of smoking, we can see the miracle of the body's adaptive mechanism at work.

Smoking drastically interferes with the body's utilization of one of our most important nutrients, vitamin C. The average smoker has close to one third less vitamin C in his body than a nonsmoker. The lack of vitamin C in our body affects the health of our gums, our susceptibility to colds, affects the production of collagen (the glue that helps build the cells of our body) and quite possibly contributes to the premature wrinkling of facial skin.

Researchers are now finding that many of the substances in cigarette smoke combine with other components in the smoke to create new and even more harmful materials. There are still many new discoveries yet to come regarding the effects of cigarette smoke.

In the movies (and in real life) when people close the garage door, turn on the car engine and wait in the front seat to die, they end their life by a method called *carbon monoxide poisoning.* The reason this is such an effective way to die is that the hemoglobin in the blood which carries life-giving oxygen to the cells of the body combines better with carbon monoxide than oxygen. So within a short amount of time hemoglobin is carrying deadly carbon monoxide in rather large amounts to all points of the body. The cells quickly become asphyxiated and die for lack of oxygen. This same carbon monoxide is also one of the main components of cigarette smoke. Most smokers actively engage at least 6 percent of their hemoglobin in carbon monoxide transport. Along with every other effect smoking has on the body, each cigarette severely limits your intake of vital oxygen. Nicotine is one of *the* most lethal substances known to man. It is incorporated into certain powerful insecticides, and one tiny drop of nicotine injected into the bloodstream can kill you in a matter of minutes. The smoke in one cigarette contains only a fraction of a drop of nicotine, about 0.5 milligrams.

One of the reasons we continue to smoke is the quick and temporary feeling of stimulation that occurs as a result of nicotine poisoning. Because this elation is based on chemical stimulation it is temporary and followed by an equal amount of destimulation or depression. In creating this "up," nicotine works on the sympathetic and the central nervous systems. Next, it stimulates the adrenal glands to give off epinephrine, the chemical that gives runners that wonderful feeling of exhilaration they experience during peak running ventures. Unfortunately when the epinephrine is squeezed out of the adrenals by nicotine (and not by physical exertion) it is quickly countered by feelings of fatigue and minor depression. While all this chemistry is going on, nicotine does not neglect the liver. It forces the liver to pump out a healthy supply of glycogen, better known as sugar. This sugar gets your muscles all excited. But by the time they get around to exploiting this new thrust of fuel the artificial stimulation has deserted them. This sudden thrust of stimulation in combination with all the other chemical chaos brought on by nicotine accounts for the physical sensations caused by smoking.

On a less chemical and more physical level, smoking rearranges the structure and functioning of the protective mechanisms of the lungs, causing them eventually to turn in on themselves, becoming their own worst enemy. This is a somewhat slow yet thorough process.

Each cigarette causes irritation to the entire respiratory tract. Generally the lungs have a system for responding to such occasional irritation by particulate matter or smoke. The cells lining the bronchial tubes secrete a very sticky substance that acts like flypaper to trap dust and particles. This sticky material, known as mucous, is moved throughout the respiratory system and out of the body by tiny moving hairs. They transport the mucous and dust up to the throat, where it is coughed out or to the stomach. Not only does smoking create a lot of dirt for the lungs but it eventually destroys these helpful little cilia. The lungs are left defenseless against the ravages of smoke, dust and grime. The protective mechanisms that remain in the lungs continue to pump out mucous in a last-chance effort to prevent further injury to the lungs. Without the cilia the respiratory system can literally drown in excess unciliated mucous. The mucous begins to build up in the bronchi, and its attempt to get out of the body results in that irritating habit known as smokers' cough.

While cigarette smoke undermines the functions of the lungs and overwhelms the circulatory system, its destructive effects extend to the heart. Smoking can foster a condition known as atherosclerosis, in which the blood vessels become congested, making it harder for the blood to pass through. Thus the heart has to pump harder and harder, putting an increased strain on its mechanism. After each cigarette, the heart rate tends to increase just a bit, along with a complementary increase in blood pressure.

Mothers tend to be quite influential on the development of their offspring. Studies are now finding that the mother's influence extends even before birth, while the child is still being formed. Women who smoke deliver more babies that die within the first month than those who don't smoke. In addition they have more unsuccessful pregnancies, more still births, more premature babies as well as smaller babies. Most of these complications are attributed to the carbon monoxide taken up by blood. The mother deprives the unborn child of essential oxygen during its development. Smokers' babies accumulate nicotine and other components of smoking during the fetal period. And the long-range effects of these substances are just now being studied for the first time.

The more cigarettes you smoke, the more likely you will experience a decrease in endurance, stamina and life expectancy. On the whole, the death rate for men and women who smoke is 70 percent higher than the rate for nonsmokers. Each year millions and millions of working hours are lost because of illness related to smoking. If these figures were translated into the amount of tangible goods people sacrifice yearly because of their involvement in smoking they would realize that it is better to be greedy and healthy than to be deprived and sick. The National Clearinghouse for Smoking and Health has stated that because people smoke there are 111 million more chronic cases of illness yearly in this country.

Nothing sends chills up and down the spines of people everywhere than the word *cancer*. In fact, cancer has become so prevalent that it is one of the great silent epidemics of this century, striking one out of every four Americans.

With cancer, the body gets confused as to what it's supposed to do in order to maintain a normal existence. The cells go crazy, losing their sense of allegiance, and begin multiplying and attacking nearly everything in sight. This

overthrow of cellular order by guerrilla cells results in new
coalitions that continue to make ever-increasingly successful
terrorist strikes at major and minor outposts throughout the
body. Lung cancer is one of the most deadly and
unfortunately prevalent forms of cancer. Newly emerging
cancer cells tend to get their start in the lungs because of the
rich supply of blood and lymph. Once a cancer starts in the
lungs, the continual supply of blood and lymph can carry it
anywhere throughout the body. Thus a cancer starting in the
lungs is more than likely to end up elsewhere in the body.
To complicate matters further, the presence of cancer often
goes undetected until it has become well established within
the body. The symptoms tend to be somewhat ordinary—
maybe just a cough or a little sore spot in the chest. But then
these are accepted as standard for anyone smoking.

Once cancer gets started in the body, the odds are not
very good for stopping it. You can have your lungs taken out
piece by piece, have your cells destroyed and lose your hair
through chemotherapy or get bombarded with tissue-
destroying radiation—and the chances are still pretty good
that you're not going to make it. Without sounding alarmist,
the American Cancer Society recommendation on "How to
Help Protect Against Lung Cancer" is simple: "Don't smoke.
If you do smoke, stop." As an encouraging aside, it has been
found that smokers who quit before cancer finds its way into
their bodies stand a good chance of reducing their risks to the
level faced by the nonsmoking population. Ten years after
quitting, ex-smokers are only very slightly more likely than
nonsmokers to develop the dread disease.

Along with lung cancer there are several other minor
forms of cancer that occur because of smoking. Cancer of the
larynx can destroy the mechanism we use for talking and in
some cases requires surgical removal of the larynx and the
construction of a permanent opening in the neck. Cancer of
the mouth, or oral cancer, can also require disfiguring
surgery, but fortunately it is one cancer that can be readily
seen and thus treated. To reduce the chances of contracting
mouth and throat cancers, smokers should also change other
habits. Many smokers enjoy their cigarettes the most when

drinking coffee or alcohol. It just so happens that alcohol has the ability to increase the penetration capacity of the cancerous substances present in cigarette smoke. This means that late evenings of bar-hopping and cigarette smoking create a powerful synergistic effect, greatly increasing your chances of getting cancer of the esophagus. Incidentally, smoking also fosters a great deal of cancer both in the bladder and the kidney.

■ STOPPING SMOKING

Stopping smoking is not the traumatic event everyone makes it out to be. The first step comes when you decide to stop. Once you've decided that you no longer enjoy the benefits of smoking, it gets that much easier to quit. It's rather fascinating to watch the rituals that people create in order not to light a cigarette. They can get extremely involved in exhausting seminars, hypnosis or any number of sucking devices. Probably the best way to quit is to replace smoking with an analagous process that creates similar effects. The closest process to smoking is breathing. People tend to get terribly frightened of living life without cigarettes. They simply can't imagine having a meal or a conversation or watching television without breathing in smoke. Specific breathing exercises function as an actual physiological and psychological replacement for the needs and desires that smoking creates.

You have to prepare yourself mentally for the fact that you are about to become a nonsmoker. Although this is indeed a positive goal, many people fear reaching it. One of the attractions of smoking is that it allows us to sneak a little break in here and there during the busy day, especially if we can't just leave work to go out and play softball. In a way the act of smoking gives you permission to relax, take a break. By lighting up a cigarette you are legitimizing the fact that you are indeed taking a break, no matter how busy you really are. In less time than it takes you to find a cigarette, light up and smoke it, you can relieve any feelings of anxiety or tension and feel more refreshed just through a few seconds of breathing.

What we are going to provide you with is a series of very specific breathing exercises that will replace the physical sensations that you get from smoking and will steadily work toward increasing your lung capacity, strengthening your cardiovascular system as well as relieving and breaking up bronchial congestion that has been created by smoking. Through proper breathing you will find yourself actually not enjoying or needing smoking. As your smoking desires lessen, your overall general feelings of health and well-being will greatly improve. The results will speak for themselves.

Stopping smoking is a gradual process. If, for example, you have a cigarette about every thirty or forty minutes, just by skipping one cigarette every several hours you are already well on the way to quitting. Quitting is nothing more than just passing by, one after another, the opportunity to light a cigarette. Once you've decided that you are going to stop, consider yourself a nonsmoker, not a smoker that is trying to stop. Once you get going, especially after the first day, it's easier than you think. In this program you will replace the cigarette cravings with enhanced stamina and a renewed body. The exercises in the Stop Smoking Program are designed to achieve three main goals. The first is to provide a physiological and psychological substitute for smoking, so the exercises should be used whenever you desire a cigarette. Along with giving you an alternative to the physical action of smoking and its effects on the lungs and body, these breathing exercises will relieve anxiety and tension. Thus, after a few breaths you will not only have bypassed your craving for a cigarette but you will also be feeling much more refreshed and alert than had you smoked.

The second aspect of the program is to re-educate you in the proper use of your lungs. During this part of the program you will be increasing your chest capacity, stretching your rib cage both up and out and generally improving the effectiveness of your respiratory system. You will become aware of what it is like really to take a deep breath and how good it feels. Day by day you will be reclaiming the unused areas of your lungs. By employing the exercises given, your breathing will soon be functioning at optimum capacity. Most likely you will be so overwhelmed with the energy and enhanced breathing that you will never again give the slightest consideration to smoking.

The third goal of the program is the cleaning and regeneration of your respiratory system. Some of the exercises will begin to remove the stale air and smoke that have been trapped within your lungs. This old air prevents you from breathing fully and tends to increase your need and desire to smoke. As this air is gradually moved out from the lungs it will be replaced with a continual supply of fresh oxygen that will then be utilized to the maximum by the body. Your posture, skin color and general well-being will greatly improve. A secondary aspect of these lung-cleaning exercises is to stretch and exercise the lungs themselves. Under the stress of smoking, the lungs tend to lose their elasticity. These exercises will begin stimulating vital points within the lungs and chest so that they may become reactivated. With a minimal investment of time and energy the breathing program will not only alleviate your desire and need to smoke but will, more importantly, greatly enhance the vitality and capability of your respiratory system.

The first step in stopping smoking is learning how to breathe properly. Up until now you have been steadily decreasing the amount of oxygen your body takes in because of your smoking. Initially it may be difficult to take a deep breath. You must immediately switch over all your breathing to the total breath. (See *Total Breathing* instructions, page 00.) There are specific exercises in this program that will enable you to loosen the tightness or strain you feel in your chest every time you attempt to breathe deeply. You will find that as you begin practicing the total breath, over a very short period of time it will become the preferred and automatic form of breathing.

■ SMOKING SUBSTITUTES

These breathing exercises are designed to satisfy your cigarette cravings and replace the relaxing sensations that you get from smoking. They should be used as often as possible, and they are not habit-forming. Each time you feel the need for a cigarette, use one or a combination of the following exercises as many times as you wish. The average is about four or five times each time you need a cigarette. The *no-smoking breath* is perfect for use during the day, at the office, after dinner or whenever there is a tension build-up in the chest area that needs to be relieved. It is quite similar to smoking and functions as an acceptable replacement.

■ NO-SMOKING BREATH

1. Forcefully inhale the total breath. Breathe in as deeply as possible.
2. Hold the breath for two seconds.
3. Tilt your head slightly back and exhale through your mouth with great force. As you exhale, shape your lips into a tiny "0" so that the air has to be forced out during the exhalation. Pull in your stomach with the exhalation so that the air is really forced out. See Fig. 11.
4. After repeating this breath three or four times, finish off with a regular total breath.
5. After the initial cigarette craving has left, you may want to repeat this exercise, only a bit more gently. Often people find themselves yawning briefly after this exercise, as the body accommodates itself to a new supply of fresh oxygen.

■ RELAXATION BREATH

Although this breath is somewhat similar to the one above the release of the breath relieves different areas of stress.

1. Gently inhale the total breath.
2. Hold the breath for three seconds.
3. Clench your teeth and open your lips. Force the air out between the teeth. You will be making a hissing sound like a tea kettle.
4. Repeat four times. You may wish to vary the intensity of the exhalation and the hissing. For some people, a

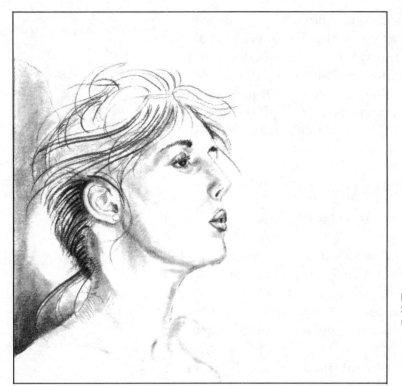

Fig. 11. No Smoking Breath, Step 3. Exhale as if you were smoking a cigarette.

slight, almost inaudible hiss is more effective than a loud forceful hiss.

5. Return to normal breathing with the total breath.

■ "AHH" BREATH

1. Gently inhale the total breath, filling the lower lungs first, then the midsection and finally the upper part of the chest.

2. Hold the breath for three seconds.

3. Open your mouth, and as you exhale the breath, release a giant sigh, making a tension-releasing "Ahh" sound. Again, remember to exhale beginning with the abdomen and gently working upward until you have released all the air.

4. Return to normal breathing with the total breath.

Experiment with all these exercises and find the one

most effective for you. Some find they accrue more benefits from mixing exercises. For example, after three repetitions of the no-smoking breath, finish your relaxation with the "ahh" breath.

■ RELEASE BREATH

The *release breath* is used as a supplementary exercise to the smoking substitutes. Its purpose is to lower anxiety levels and reinforce the effect of proper breathing. It requires a bit of mental visualization as well.

1. Close your eyes as you inhale the total breath. Imagine that you are inhaling pure relaxation. You may want to use a visual image to reinforce this concept. Imagine a soothing color such as a cool blue or picture a perfect day at the beach and breathe in that clean, slightly salty crisp air.
2. Hold for three seconds. During this period mentally gather up *all* the tensions in your body. Check your face, the muscles in your cheeks, around your eyes and especially the back of your neck and your shoulders. Scan the rest of your body for any other tensions. Get ready to breathe them out in the exhalation. Gather any remaining tension and dissolve it into the air that you now retain in your lungs.
3. Exhale through slightly rounded lips, as if you were going to whistle. As you exhale, actually feel those tensions leaving your body on a steady stream of air.
4. Inhale a complete deep total breath and exhale forcefully through an open mouth.

■ LUNG CLEANING

In general most people have faulty exhalation habits whether they smoke or not. Over the years, increasing amounts of stale air become trapped within the lungs. By continually retaining this air you restrict the lungs' ability to take in their full capacity of fresh air, thereby depriving the body of proper oxygenation. And if you smoke, you greatly increase the amount of stale air you retain. Pockets of stale air develop throughout the respiratory system which not only inhibit your natural breathing but also provide the breeding ground for various diseases and complications which affect the respiratory system and eventually the entire body.

The following set of breathing exercises is designed to extract larger and larger portions of stale dead air while increasingly ventilating the lungs. Ideally these exercises should be performed at least twice a day, in the morning before work and in the evening before dinner. You might wish to add an additional set about an hour before bed, because sleep is the time during which the lungs and the skin rid themselves of accumulated toxins.

■ LUNG STIMULATION BREATH

1. For this exercise you may stand or sit, but far superior results are achieved through standing.
2. Very slowly inhale the total breath. As you inhale, lightly pound your chest with the fingertips of both hands, moving them randomly about to cover the upper chest, breast area and the sides of the rib cage. If you find yourself coughing, decrease the pressure with which you pound.
3. Hold the breath for five seconds and gently slap the entire area of your chest with flat open hands.
4. Exhale through rounded lips.
5. Inhale the total breath.
6. Retain for five seconds.
7. Now gently rub or caress your chest, upper chest, breast area and the sides of your rib cage with flat open palms.
8. Exhale through rounded lips.
9. Inhale the total breath.
10. Retain for five seconds.
11. Exhale through rounded lips.

This exercise will stimulate both the muscles and the cells of the respiratory system. The light pounding or percussion will begin to ease and break up the congestion that prevents you from breathing deeper. When you finish the lung stimulation exercise, your entire chest area will tingle and your breathing will be freer and easier. By activating the cells, you increase their strength and start to fortify their ability to begin regenerating important lung tissue.

■ RETAINED BREATH

1. Stand erect.
2. Inhale the total breath.
3. Hold the breath as long as possible. (This does not mean retaining the breath until you are dizzy and about to pass out.) Start by holding this breath for about twenty seconds, then gradually work your way upward, adding another five or ten seconds whenever you feel comfortable in doing so.
4. Exhale forcefully through your mouth. As you finish the exhalation, pull your stomach in again and you will find that there is a second exhalation. Squeeze this last bit of air out of your lungs. In this way you will be continually cleaning out the reserve air that accumulates with each inhalation.
5. Return to total breathing. Repeat the entire exercise three times. This exercise strengthens and helps increase the elasticity of the respiratory muscles, as well as stretching out the lungs and the chest. By forcefully exhaling two times you remove residual air that prevents the body from being properly oxygenated.

■ PISTON BREATH

This breath furthers the elimination of stale useless air from the lungs.

1. Sit comfortably erect in a chair or on the floor.
2. Inhale the total breath.
3. Quickly exhale the breath through the nose by contracting the stomach as far in as possible. See Fig. 12.

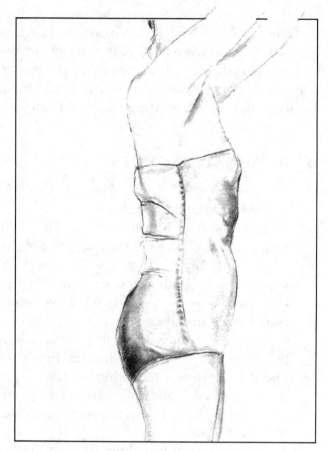

Fig. 12. Piston Breath, Step 3.
Pull the stomach in to exhale.

4. As you release the stomach, simultaneously take in another total breath. See Fig. 13.

5. Repeat this inhalation and forceful exhalation ten times in a row. Your stomach should be rapidly moving in and out like a piston, and your breath should sound like a choo-choo train gradually picking up speed.

6. After ten times inhale the total breath. Hold for five seconds and exhale.

■ LUNG ENHANCEMENT

Most of us are habitually poor breathers not only because we don't know how to breathe correctly but because our lungs through improper breathing, poor posture and stress tend to

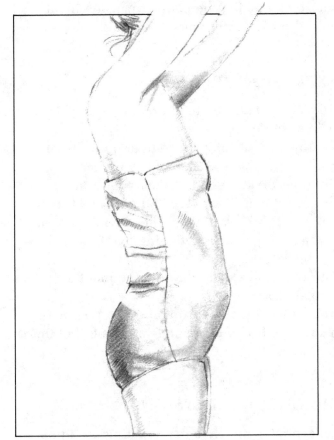

Fig. 13. Piston Breath, Step 4. Push the stomach out to begin the next inhalation.

lose their natural tone and elasticity. In addition, the rib cage lazily refuses to expand itself to its maximum capacity. With poor breathing our lungs become filled with stagnant air, the intercostal muscles surrounding the ribs do not get their proper exercise and our breathing then becomes increasingly shallow and restricted to the upper areas of the lungs. The following exercises are designed to stretch and expand the rib cage while simultaneously filling the lungs to their full capacity. In this way, deeper breathing will become more comfortable and more automatic. As you begin to enhance your breathing, cigarettes will become increasingly unsatisfying. The *chest expansion breath* will progressively fill the chest cavity with increasing amounts of air. It will also stretch out the sternum and lift the rib cage, facilitating deep natural breathing. Incidentally, the chest expansion breath is also quite beneficial for improving one's posture.

■ CHEST EXPANSION BREATH

1. Stand erect and inhale the total breath.
2. Hold for five counts.
3. Lift both arms so that they are straight out in front of you at shoulder level. Now, make a fist with each hand. While holding the breath, gently swing your arms horizontally toward your back. Try and get your fists to touch as they meet in back of you. Then swing your arms to the front again. Repeat this swinging five times while still holding the breath.
4. Drop your arms and exhale through the mouth.
5. Inhale a total breath.
6. Repeat this entire procedure three times. When you finish, your lungs will feel clean and capable of holding much more air.

■ RHYTHMIC CHEST EXPANSION

This exercise concentrates mostly on stimulating the upper chest area.

1. Stand erect and inhale the total breath.
2. Hold for five seconds.
3. Bring your arms out in front of you at shoulder level and with fists clenched gently swing them horizontally toward the back. As you do so, exhale forcefully through an open mouth. See Fig. 14.
4. Breathe in through the nose as you return the arms in front of you.
5. Exhale and swing the arms to the back again.
6. Repeat this back-and-forth inhalation/exhalation routine at least ten times.

As you exhale stale air you are increasing the strength of the upper lung and its attendant muscles.

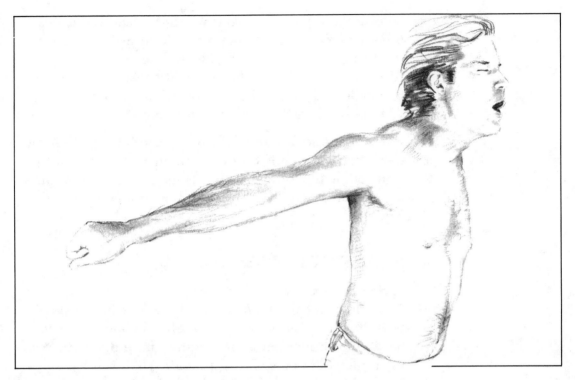

Fig. 14. Rhythmic Chest Expansion, Step 3. Exhale completely as you bring your arms back.

The *rib stretch breath* pulls up the rib cage into a position that fosters deeper breathing. The accompanying arm movement stimulates the musculature attached to the ribs.

■ RIB STRETCH BREATH

1. Inhale the total breath.
2. While holding your breath, lift your arms forward and up over your head and then backward until you have performed a circular movement. You are like a windmill catching the currents of the wind. Continue this swinging motion at least fifteen times. If at any point you feel you can't hold your breath any longer, exhale and then inhale through the nose an additional breath of air until you have reached fifteen counts.
3. Lower your hands to your sides and exhale.
4. Inhale and repeat the swinging process, only this time

reverse the direction of your windmill. Start the hands from the back, bringing them over your head to your front and again rotate them fifteen times.

5. Drop your hands to the side and exhale.

6. Inhale and exhale the total breath three times.

7. Repeat the entire process three times.

The *body stretch breath* lifts the entire body and the rib cage. The body stretch is best done upon awakening. In this way you completely oxygenate and stimulate the body while starting the day immediately with full breathing instead of a cigarette.

■ BODY STRETCH BREATH

1. Stand erect with your hands at your sides.

2. Begin to inhale the total breath. As you inhale slowly, begin to raise your arms in front of you and up over your head. As you lift your arms, begin to raise the body itself by lifting your heels off the ground. When you have finished inhaling, your arms should be straight up over your head, and all your body weight should be supported by your toes and the balls of your feet.

3. Hold for six counts.

4. Slowly bring your arms down to your sides, lower the body and exhale through your nose.

5. In normal standing position, inhale the total breath and release through the mouth.

6. Repeat the entire exercise three times.

By avoiding the temptation to smoke your next cigarette you have already gone a long way to stopping smoking. As you reach for your next cigarette remind yourself that you *have* stopped, and if you do not light this one you will be two cigarettes into being a nonsmoker. From there the number of cigarettes you don't smoke will soon surpass the number that you do.

Whenever you begin to feel tension or tightness in the chest or whenever you are about to light a cigarette, *immediately* do one of the smoking substitute breathing exercises, preferably the no-smoking breath. This will get you through that seemingly impossible period where you *"have"* to have a cigarette. In fact afterward you will feel more relaxed, more awake than you would had you had a cigarette. When next the cigarette urge calls, again use one of the smoking substitute breathing exercises. If you feel you absolutely can't wait and you must have a cigarette, make a deal with yourself that you will perform the breathing exercise *before* you have the cigarette. Repeat the no-smoking breath three or four times. Afterward pause for a minute, fold your hands and say, "I have now not smoked a total of X cigarettes since starting this program. Do I really want this cigarette?" If the answer is yes, then perform the breathing exercise one more time. And then go ahead and have your cigarette. But after the cigarette perform the breathing exercise one more time. If this one cigarette has indeed proven to be enjoyable, don't worry. This "pleasurable" sensation will definitely decrease. Above all, don't scold yourself. Tell yourself that you are not a failure and that you haven't spoiled all the good behavior you've worked so hard to achieve. The rationalization that since you've had this one cigarette you've started smoking again and you may as well go back to smoking is utter nonsense. You have not had a setback, nor have you failed the program. After successfully not smoking a certain number of cigarettes you have only smoked *one*. That means your batting average at this point is actually quite high. You should be proud of yourself. You've done quite well. Another point to consider is that you have been smoking quite a few years and a couple of days or even half a day without cigarettes is a vast improvement. You have already made great strides toward reversing your smoking behavior. So forget about undermining your own determination to stop smoking. It's of no use, because eventually you will find breathing infinitely more satisfying than smoking.

There are very few smokers who do not really want to stop. Since this seems to be the prevalent feeling, you should feel very lucky that you have begun such a program. There is little doubt that you will achieve your goal.

The following breathing schedule is a guide that will help you through that crucial first week of not smoking. Since each person has individual needs, feel free to make exercise substitutions or rearrange the schedule to your preferences.

■ STOP-SMOKING BREATHING SCHEDULE

DAY ONE

1. Upon arising do the body stretch once, followed by two repetitions of the lung stimulation.
2. Remember to breathe only with the total breath.
3. If you usually have your first cigarette after breakfast, substitute the no-smoking breath.
4. During the day whenever you customarily reach for a cigarette or you start thinking of cigarettes excessively, pause for a moment and do three repetitions of the no-smoking breath.
5. During any low period of the day when you feel stale or overly taxed, perform the chest expansion three times.
6. During your lunch hour try to get outside for a walk and continue total breathing.
7. When you get home do the chest expansion and two repetitions of the retained breath.
8. After dinner and during the evening, especially if you watch television, remember to use the no-smoking breath or the "ahh" breath to release the tensions of the day and relieve any feelings of anxieties about not smoking.
9. Just before you go to sleep, lie in your bed, close your eyes and do several rounds of the release breath.

DAY TWO

1. Upon arising, repeat the body stretch two times, followed by two repetitions of the lung stimulation breath and two repetitions of the rib stretch.
2. Throughout the day continue to breathe the total breath.
3. Remember to use any of the cigarette substitute breaths whenever necessary.

4. If again the pressure of not smoking gets too intense, practice the retained breath three or four times.

5. Lunch: body stretch.

6. Before dinner: three repetitions of chest expansion, three of lung stimulation.

7. Evening: five repetitions of relaxation breath.

8. Bedtime: release breath.

DAY THREE

1. Upon awakening: three body stretch and three lung stimulation.

2. After breakfast: retained breath.

3. During the day: cigarette substitute breaths, especially the no-smoking breath.

4. Lunch: chest expansion.

5. Before dinner: rib stretch three times, retained breath three times.

6. Evening: three relaxation breaths followed by three repetitions of the "ahh" breath.

7. Bedtime: release breath.

DAY FOUR

1. Upon awakening: three body stretch and four rhythmic chest expansion.

2. After breakfast: no-smoking breath.

3. During the day: total breathing and cigarette substitute breaths as needed.

4. Lunch: three rib stretches.

5. Before dinner: four lung stimulations and three chest expansions.

6. Evening: three retained breaths.

7. Bedtime: release breath.

DAY FIVE (THE TURNING POINT)

1. Upon awakening: three chest expansions and four lung stimulations.

2. After breakfast: three retained breaths.

3. During the day: total breathing and cigarette substitute breaths as needed.

4. Lunch: lung stimulation three times.

5. Before dinner: three "ahh" breaths and three retained breaths.

6. Evening: "ahh" breath three times and no-smoking breath as needed.

7. Bedtime: release breath.

Day Six

1. Upon awakening: three rib stretches, three rhythmic chest expansions and one lung stimulation.

2. After breakfast: no-smoking breath.

3. During the day: total breathing and cigarette substitute breaths as needed.

4. Lunch: rib stretch three times.

5. Before dinner: three body stretches and three rhythmic chest expansions.

6. Evening: relaxation breath three times.

7. Bedtime: release breath.

Day Seven

1. Upon awakening: body stretch three times, rhythmic chest expansion three times.

2. After breakfast: no-smoking breath.

3. During the day: total breathing and cigarette substitute.

4. Lunch: retained breath.

5. Before dinner: rhythmic chest expansion and lung stimulation.

6. Evening: "ahh" breath.

7. Bedtime: release breath.

It's quite useful to make an index card daily to keep with you regarding that particular day's breathing program. You might wish to fill it out just as they have been listed here. On the back of the card, for your own satisfaction, keep a record of achievement, of how many cigarettes you have *not* smoked. For every cigarette that you do not smoke by using one of the substitute breathing exercises, make a plus sign on the back of the card. For every cigarette that you somehow manage to get into your mouth and smoke, make a minus sign. Whenever you are weakening in your temptation to smoke you might wish to review your achievements before you give in. At the end of the day, before bed and before you leave in the morning, review your progress and vow that you will meet or surpass the past day's progress.

6

BEAUTY PROGRAM

MANY PEOPLE THINK of fashionable
clothes and stylish haircuts as the keys to beauty, and it is
true that they contribute to overall attractiveness. Every
culture has developed important ways of making the body
more attractive, including the use of makeup in ancient Egypt
and the latest New York fashions. But real beauty must
radiate from the body itself. A man or woman who sparkles
with physical health and vitality will look beautiful no matter
what he or she wears.

Beauty has to do with a certain calmness and confidence
about oneself as well as the health and quality of the hair,
skin and eyes. There are countless preparations on the market
that can externally do a great deal of good in the maintenance
of the hair, skin and eyes. But true health and true beauty
must come from within the body. All the cosmetics in the
world can do little to remedy the ravages of oxygen-depleted
skin. An abundant supply of oxygen and blood to the head is
crucial for the maintenance and attractiveness of our faces.
Without adequate oxygen the skin begins to sag and

accumulate wastes, thus aging rapidly; the eyes lose their sparkle, and the hair becomes straggly and dull. Poor circulation can only minimally remove the accumulated cellular wastes from the head region. Through proper breathing and improved circulation we can greatly enhance both our internal health and our external appearance.

Correct posture is often considered to be an indication of proper breeding, but more importantly it is a contributor to the overall health of the body. Poor posture also affects the spinal cord. The spine or backbone is the major conductor of nerve messages through the body. Its health is critical to the proper functioning of all sensory and regulatory organs. If we stoop or sag we interfere with the optimum functioning of the spine and the nerve messages it sends. A healthy spine definitely contributes to our health and longevity. Old age and inflexibility both in body and mind often occur when there is a stiff and unbending spine. As the spine loses its flexibility the major conduits of nerve energy become stagnant. Thus that attractive glowing vitality that represents health and beauty begins to degenerate. Physical therapists insist that you will stay healthy and young as long as your spine is flexible. Through proper posture and correct breathing you can maintain a flexible spine and also project a greater image of physical self-worth.

How we stand and how we sit affects how we breathe. If the body is slumped over, the shoulders become rounded and the rib cage collapses, giving the lungs no room to expand. Our breathing then becomes restricted to only the upper area of the lungs. Notice the difference in your ability to breathe deeply when you are slumped over a desk and when you are sitting erectly, giving the lungs a chance for maximum expansion. And the reverse is equally as true; how we breathe directly affects our posture. It is virtually impossible to have poor posture if we are breathing properly. The very process of total breathing requires that the spine be erect and the shoulders properly aligned.

Poor posture inhibits the flow of oxygen throughout the body. With less oxygen taken in, every cell in the body then becomes undernourished and hungry for fresh oxygen. Of paramount importance is the circulation to the head area. Because of gravity, blood carrying oxygen naturally has to work harder to get up above the heart into the head. When poor posture interferes with circulation it also affects the skin, hair and eyes. Posture also tends to be an unconscious expression of the body. Through posture we reflect our moods, our mental states. Lack of confidence, fear, poor self-esteem are accurately portrayed in the way we stand. Whereas at those times when we are feeling proud of our accomplishments, full of self-satisfaction and energy, the body naturally tends to hold itself with pride. It is not possible to maintain a good carriage and feel depressed or out of sorts. Incidentally, next time you are at a party or out in public, notice who catches your eye and why. Aside from high fashion, people with good posture and a sense of ease with their bodies are always extremely attractive.

Most of us think of posture in the stiff, militaristic fashion, shoulders back and chest out. This is a rigid and nonfunctional form of posture that is great for statues but not for human beings on the move. Essentially posture is a method for keeping the body properly aligned. Above all, good posture must be comfortable. One of the easiest methods for insuring good posture is to imagine that there is a string attached to the top of your head gently pulling your entire body erect. As the string is pulled upward your chin is at a right angle with the floor, your breast bone naturally pulls back, your pelvis rotates slightly forward so that your buttocks pull in and your stomach lies flat. You should feel your weight evenly distributed along the foot from the toes to the ball and the heel. When people stand "straight" in the conventional sense, a small arch develops in the lower back. Eventually this can lead to chronic lower back pain. The rotating of the pelvis can help correct this little arch in the small of the back. By rotating the pelvis forward and pulling in the buttocks, you will feel your lower back flatten. This is the comfortable posture you should maintain at all times.

Many people with poor posture walk with their chins tilted slightly downward and their shoulders curved forward. This posture restricts the breath to the upper lungs. With your chin slightly pointing to the ground, take a deep inhalation. Most likely the breath will make a wheezing sound as it enters the nose. Your lungs will become partially filled just to the breast area. Now, look straight ahead with your chin parallel to the ground and inhale. The breath enters the body in a smooth quiet stream with no obstruction and your lungs become completely filled. Improved posture and correct breathing increase the blood flow throughout the body. It also affects the tone and radiance of the skin. As you continue to improve the oxygen content of the body, your cheeks will achieve that legendary rosiness without applying any color from a tube. Your whole face will take on a vibrant radiance that speaks of good health. The energy level of the body and the clarity of your thoughts will also improve.

One of the major problems with telling somebody to just stand up straight is the difficulty of properly demonstrating the experience of good posture. In the army when they tell you "shoulders back" they do not teach you how to let the body fall into its own proper posture. The *posture stretch* combines breathing and stretching to set the body into a correct posture.

■ POSTURE STRETCH

1. Inhale the total breath.
2. Raise both arms out in front of you and extend them up over your head. Your hands should be pointing straight up to the ceiling.
3. Holding the breath, raise yourself up on your toes and reach for the ceiling. You should feel the stretch running from down your arms, shoulder blades, chest, sides and especially at the abdomen. Hold for ten seconds.
4. Lower your heels back to the ground.
5. As you exhale through the nostrils, bring your arms out to the sides and let them float down. This will provide a nice stretch for the upper chest area.
6. Repeat the exercise three times.

You will feel the chest lifted and resting above the abdomen. The head will float nicely centered on the neck and without tension. Try to retain this comfortable posture throughout the day. If you feel your muscles sagging, perform the posture stretch whenever necessary to reinstate proper posture.

■ POSTURE BREATH

1. Stand with your feet about six inches apart and your eyes looking straight ahead.
2. Exhale.
3. Inhale the total breath. As you inhale pull up the breast bone.
4. Holding the breath, tighten and pull in the buttocks. Now, without exhaling, inhale again.
5. Hold for ten seconds.
6. As you exhale maintain the posture you have achieved.
7. Repeat three times.

The posture breath provides important realignment for the spine and shoulders of the body. Often when standing our buttocks and stomach curve outward. This throws the body out of synch while laying the foundation for future lower back problems. The tightening of the buttocks provides exercise for that neglected area. If you maintain this posture after exhaling you will find breathing becomes much easier. With proper posture the body becomes much more alive and awake. Your movements take on an air of grace and style. It is a good idea to practice the posture breath the first thing in the morning. If you are in the habit of sloppy posture, practice the breath several times a day until proper posture becomes second nature.

The *swing breath* increases the oxygen supply to the head and helps remove toxic wastes that can cause cellular aging.

■ SWING BREATH

1. Standing, spread your legs about three feet apart.
2. Raise your arms above your head, lifting up the entire body, inhale a total breath, hold for three or four seconds.

3. With your hands guiding you down, slowly lower the trunk of the body. Exhale as you bend over.

4. Let your head and hands hang for fifteen seconds.

5. Now slowly raise your body back up. As you inhale the total breath bring your arms up over your head, hold for three or four seconds.

6. Continue with step 3.

7. Repeat this exercise three times.

Excess weight is one of the major beauty and health problems in America. In part it has a great deal to do with the kind of food we eat as well as the amount we eat. Yet being overweight is also directly tied to the way we breathe and how much we breathe. A great deal of the digestive process is dependent on oxygen for its fuel. The digestion of food requires enormous amounts of energy in order to break down the complex food molecules and transform them into usable substances that can feed the body. As the body takes in less oxygen through improper breathing, metabolic processes occur at a much slower rate and often food is insufficiently digested. This means that there is a greater opportunity for the food to become fat. Then as the body's weight increases this puts a handicap on the functioning of the entire respiratory system. As this cycle continues, breathing becomes increasingly difficult and the body continues to metabolize food at a slower pace. This progresses to the stage that we often see in obese people who must struggle for every breath. Because of the enormous strain on the body their breathing becomes quick and shallow. As the body continues to labor for air, the intake of food becomes greater because the body is unable to digest properly the food that is eaten. The body then seeks to acquire its necessary energy from more food. Thus the cycle continues on and on, virtually intensifying both hunger and overeating patterns.

By fully utilizing and digesting all the food you take in, you naturally reduce the need for increased servings and feedings. Your craving for starches and sweets tends to decrease. With proper breathing the body also receives the added benefit of "oxygen nutrition" which contributes a great deal to reducing hunger. By emphasizing breathing in any weight-reduction program, you will find your need for food greatly decreasing. Rather than taking endless numbers of "reducing pills," which interfere with the normal metabolic functioning of the body, or by following severe starvation diets, which may upset blood-sugar levels and cause dizziness, weakness and irritability, it is much more logical and efficient simply to help the body thoroughly utilize the food eaten. Breathing can help reactivate much of the body's sluggish metabolism that has occurred because of excess weight and excess food.

In this program we want to stimulate the body and activate the digestive process through breathing. Remember, in any of the breathing exercises make sure you exhale as fully as possible. The body normally retains a small reserve of oxygen after each exhalation. However, poor breathers tend to accumulate larger portions of stale air. This retained air takes up important lung area which prevents the proper inflow of oxygen. Thus, to receive maximum benefit from any breathing exercise, thorough exhalation is as important as deep inhalation. With time and practice, deep and thorough inhalation and exhalation will become automatic.

The first thing we want to do is rediscover the muscles of the stomach. As it is, most people breathe from the chest up, but overweight individuals somehow manage to breathe in an even smaller area of the upper lungs which totally neglects the use of the rib cage and the diaphragm. *Total breathing for the stomach* will increase your awareness of the stomach and help curb excessive eating.

■ TOTAL BREATHING FOR THE STOMACH

1. Lying on your back, place your hands just below the belly button. This is the area that you want to fill with air first.
2. Slowly begin to inhale through your nose. Start the breath as low as possible. As you inhale, push out the lower stomach to accommodate the air and watch your hands rise with the inhalation. Let the air begin to rise

up higher by allowing the rib cage to expand both outward and upward. Finally the breath should fill the chest area above.

3. Hold the breath for a count of seven.

4. With your hands still on your stomach, exhale in the same order that you inhaled. Let the diaphragm (the area where your hands are resting) recoil, pushing the breath out. As the exhalation continues, watch your hands fall, followed by the lowering of the rib cage and chest area.

5. At the end of the exhalation, pull in your abdomen three more times for three quick additional exhalations of excess air. Not only does this create more room for incoming oxygen but gives the stomach itself as well as the abdominal muscles a bit of gentle exercise and stimulation.

6. Repeat the inhalation, making sure that you follow the proper sequence of stomach first, then rib cage and finally chest expansion. With each succeeding inhalation, try to get the breath to expand lower and lower areas of the abdomen. You will be amazed at how far down your breath can extend. By continually increasing the depth of the inhalation you are toning unused yet important abdominal muscles. Not only will this begin to firm the appearance of your stomach but it will facilitate the digestive process.

7. Repeat ten times.

Practice total breathing for the stomach once or twice a day, always on an empty stomach. Do ten sets of total breathing for the stomach at each session. The results will be felt internally as well as expressed externally. The body will feel less sluggish, more alive and less dependent on food as a source of stimulation and diversion. Our meals will become times for refueling the body, not escapist diversions or unnecessary cravings.

Many people are constantly concerned with the exterior appearance of their stomach. If they reversed that concern and became more aware of the appearance of the inside of the stomach, then the outside would take care of itself. One merely has to take a quick walk down the street to see the ravages of neglect that we allow ourselves to fall into. Through a combination of lack of fitness and poor dietary habits we have become a race of big bellies. Large stomachs have for some reason become the trademark of advanced civilization. Everyone we know is always trying to lose a little weight. Good posture and total breathing for the stomach can contribute toward the reduction of excess around the stomach. By standing correctly the stomach muscles are never given the opportunity to sag or become lax. With every total breath we take we strengthen those abdominal muscles most prone to sag.

Many of us need a little additional work around the stomach from time to time. The *tightening breath* is a simple exercise that can be done anytime, anywhere. Indeed, it should be practiced as often as possible throughout the day. It is easily done while sitting in the office or driving the car and helps combat that extra stomach that comes from periods of extended sitting. The tightening breath gently works the girdle area of the stomach through strong exhalations. Aside from toning up the exterior of the stomach, the tightening breath encourages the natural peristaltic action of the stomach, thus enhancing digestion and improving the utilization of food.

■ **TIGHTENING BREATH**

1. Sitting in a chair, slowly inhale a total breath for six counts.

2. Hold for three counts.

3. Exhale completely through the nose. After the exhalation, contract the stomach by quickly pulling it as far back into the body as possible. Without inhaling, let the stomach snap back out and contract it again; repeat one more time. With this last contraction pull the stomach muscle in and pull it up into the rib cage. Repeat this lifting motion three times.

4. Again, inhale for six counts. Now, repeat the entire procedure three times.

At first it may be a bit difficult to perform all the contractions and lifts on just one exhalation. Start slowly at first. Within a very short time you will be able to do it easily. This contraction/lifting motion strengthens the diaphragm as well as the muscles that hold the external stomach in place. If you find it hard to perform the contractions, this is just an indication of how out of shape you indeed are. With a little practice and patience you will be fit in no time.

Another exercise for toning up the appearance of our stomach is the *abdominal lift*.

■ ABDOMINAL LIFT

1. Standing with your feet about eighteen inches apart, slightly bend your knees as if you were riding a horse. Place your hands on your upper thighs.
2. Exhale completely. Contract your stomach, pulling it in. Pause for a second and then pull up.
3. Hold the stomach in for two seconds and release.
4. Repeat the contraction in and up for five times. Each day add another contraction until you work your way up to twenty.
5. Release the stomach and inhale a total breath.
6. Exhale and repeat the five contractions.
7. Repeat the entire exercise three times.

Along with our incessant concern with the appearance of our stomachs is our concern with diet. Everyone is always dieting. If it's not grapefruit, it's protein or macrobiotics. But it's always something. It seems that people are chronic dieters. Careful consideration of what we eat is indeed important. However, the constant change from one diet to the next may confuse the internal workings of the body. Persistant dieters know exactly, calorie for calorie, what they eat, yet know virtually nothing about how they eat. All they know is that they usually eat too much. There are few people who eat slowly, thoroughly chewing their food.

Contrary to what most people think, digestion does not occur only in the stomach. It begins in the mouth, with thorough chewing and chemical breakdown of the food by the saliva. Actually, saliva is one of the most important aspects of good digestion. If people chewed their food properly a great deal of stomach problems and improper digestion would be avoided. By chewing the food thoroughly you greatly reduce the work load of the stomach. You might want to experiment with chewing slowly and see how it affects your hunger. For example, eat dinner at your regular pace and the next evening make sure that you take only one reasonably sized bite at a time and chew it completely until it has been well masticated into tiny bits. You will find that by chewing slowly you alleviate your hunger with much less food. One of the problems of chronic dieters is that they are so hungry and wound up from their day that when they sit down they attack their food. Food that is gulped in this manner does not give the stomach an opportunity to send a relay signal to the brain, to let the brain know that it is full. Instead we have an insatiable hunger throughout the evening that is impossible to satisfy. It takes about twenty minutes after eating for this signal to reach the brain. In order to avoid this problem and to improve our digestion, it is important that we relax just before our meal and that we take our time during the meal. By relaxing, we will eat slower, enjoy our meal more and eat less.

A good way to release the tensions of the day and relax just before a meal is through the *sigh breath*. This breath quickly gathers up the various pressures from the day and releases them all at once.

■ **SIGH BREATH**

1. Sitting down comfortably, deeply inhale the total breath.
2. Hold for ten counts.
3. Place your hands on your knees and lean slightly forward. Open your mouth widely and exhale the entire breath in one gigantic sigh that sounds like one long "ahhh."

4. Repeat three times or four times before any meal but especially when you feel rushed or tense before eating.

The tradition of an after-dinner cup of coffee or a cigarette is to relieve the fullness that follows a big meal and to provide that spark of stimulation while the body is in the process of digestion. Many of us unconsciously take a deep breath after the meal to signal that we are fully satisfied. In this way the body takes in additional oxygen to help fuel the digestive process. After dinner you may wish to take a few slow total breaths to recharge the body. Digestion is an extremely energy-consuming process. That sleepiness you feel after a meal is a result of all the energy being poured into the digestive process. It requires a healthy supply of blood and oxygen to digest your meal properly. For additional oxygen after a meal, use the *after-dinner breath.*

■ AFTER-DINNER BREATH

1. Tip your head back slightly and inhale through the nose.
2. Let the air fill as much of the lungs as possible.
3. Hold for three counts.
4. As you exhale through the nose, slowly bring the head back into its regular position.
5. Repeat this breath until you feel more comfortable and less "stuffed."

Again, watch the way you eat. Many people inhale their food. That is, with each bite they take in a breath through the mouth. This impedes digestion and leaves food lying around waiting to be turned into fat. When you eat, place the food in the mouth; do not suck it off the fork or spoon. This swallowed air leads to gastric distress. In order to slow down your eating pace it is a good idea to inhale the total breath after you have swallowed each mouthful. This gives the stomach sufficient time to signal the brain when it has had enough food. If you should feel discomfort after the meal, it may be due to inhaled air that you gulped with the meal. Deep, full exhalations can often clear the lungs of the additional air that is causing so much discomfort. Try the *after-dinner breath II*.

■ AFTER-DINNER BREATH II

1. Lean forward just the slightest bit and slowly exhale as much air through the mouth as possible without straining. Do not contract the stomach. The lips should be just slightly parted, not wide open. See Fig. 15.
2. Now, gently take in a slow, deep total breath.
3. Hold for three seconds.
4. Then lean forward again and exhale gently through the mouth.
5. Repeat two or three times to alleviate any fullness from the meal.

Not only are the eyes our most important sensory organ; they also relay to the observer a great deal of information about our state of health and personality. Bright, attractive eyes have an almost magnetic charm for others. They speak of an individual who is vitally alive with a sense of purpose. Not only do the eyes see, but they can also help others see us. Though far from an exact science, one can gain an intuitive sense of another individual merely by observing his or her eyes and the qualities they emanate. Very few of us know the information our eyes reveal. If used properly they can communicate emotions and feelings more powerfully and immediately than words. Our eyes can express the range of emotions from anger to love to understanding. By exercising the muscles of your eyes you can greatly contribute to their continued vitality and functioning.

■ EYE BREATH I

1. As you inhale the total breath, look straight upward, without moving your head, as if you were looking into your forehead.
2. Hold the eyes in this position and the breath for a count of ten.

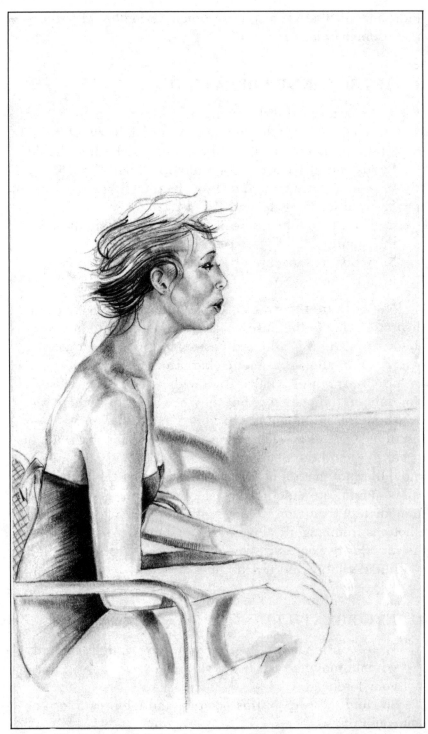

Fig. 15. After Dinner Breath II, Step 1. Lean forward and gently exhale the breath through slightly rounded lips.

3. As you quickly exhale, look straight down as if you were looking at your tongue, without moving your head.
4. Hold for ten counts.
5. Repeat eye movement ten times.

■ **EYE BREATH II**

1. As you inhale the total breath, look to the far right with both eyes without moving the head.
2. Hold the eyes in this position and the breath for a count of ten.
3. As you quickly exhale, look to the far left for a count of ten.
4. Hold for ten counts.
5. Repeat each eye movement ten times.

Most of us are horrified of being confronted with bad breath. We take great pains to avoid its occurrence with lots of mint toothpaste, green mouthwash, gum and little drops from little bottles. Odor from the mouth usually has little to do with the food we eat except in obvious examples such as garlic and onions. Very few people realize that their breath may be offensive to others because they are exhaling stale air that has been sitting around in the lungs for some time. As with any condition, prevention is often more effective than the cure. Full exhalations can do a great deal toward eliminating the unpleasant stale air from our lungs.

■ **FULL EXHALATION**

1. Sitting down with your hands on your knees, lean forward slightly and exhale as fully as possible through the mouth.
2. Still leaning slightly forward, inhale the total breath through the nose. Hold for ten counts.
3. Open your mouth widely and exhale the breath with three full contractions of the diaphragm muscle. The last exhalation should sound as if you are totally out of air.

This exercise should be done first thing in the morning and once in the evening. It can also be done just before important meetings. Aside from helping clear the lungs of

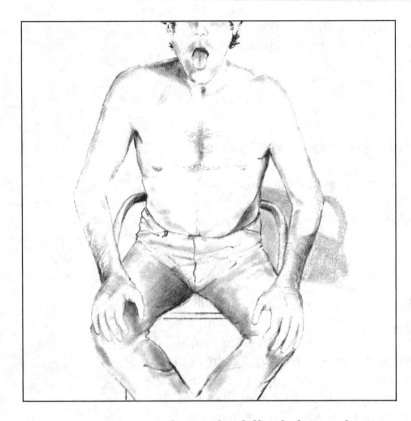

Fig. 16. Face Breath, Step 3. Look straight ahead, raise your eyebrows, stick out your tongue and exhale.

stale air, the *full exhalation* does a great deal toward promoting deeper, more thorough oxygenation of the body.

The *face breath* provides a good stretch for the throat and jaw line, the area around the eyes and the scalp.

■ FACE BREATH

1. Sitting in a chair, lean forward and place your hands on your knees.

2. Inhale the total breath through the nose.

3. As you exhale the breath, let the mouth drop wide open, stick out the tongue as far as possible and stretch your eyebrows as high up as they will go. Now exhale fully through the mouth. See Fig. 16.

4. Repeat three times.

The face breath provides important stretching and toning for those areas of the face. It also releases the tension that tends to accumulate in the various areas of the face.

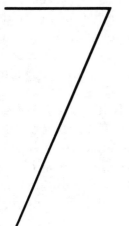

SLEEP
PROGRAM

SLEEP IS ONE OF the most
mysterious states of existence. Bizarre imagery floats in front
of our eyes and for about seven hours we remain oblivious to
the outside world. Many people consider sleeping a waste of
valuable time. They would love to eliminate sleep entirely
from their schedule and just be able to work and play twenty-
four hours a day. What these people do not realize is that
sleep is as important as any activity we do during the day.
Sleep provides us with a certain sort of physiological and
psychological shelter in which we can regenerate our bodies
and our minds. Through sleep we renew ourselves,
reorganize our energies and prepare ourselves for activity.

Sleep deprivation can produce a variety of physiological
and mental changes. Both the length of time and the way we
sleep ultimately affect both our personalities and our
physiological well-being. Extreme changes in sleep habits,
either by increasing or decreasing the amount of sleep that
we get, could be symptomatic of changes in emotional and/or
physiological health.

When deprived of sleep over extended periods of time, every aspect of our lives becomes drastically altered. Impaired concentration, uncontrollable emotions, psychic derangement, as well as general breakdown of our physical capabilities, all begin to emerge with the lack of sleep. These symptoms are also visible in poor sleepers. On the whole we tend to get too much sleep. Mostly our sleeping habits have been established by a magic yet unrealistic number of eight hours a night. If we were not so dedicated to our eight-hour sleep quota we would most likely find ourselves sleeping less yet still performing the same. On the average most of us can cut an hour or two off our sleep schedule, leaving us that much more time for engaging in other satisfying waking activities. The experiment with less sleep is worthwhile. Many have found that once they become accustomed to the new routine, they have more energy and use their time more efficiently.

Sleep serves not only to rest the body and the mind but to give the body a chance to clear itself of accumulated toxins by ventilation of the body through breathing. As the body rests, the by-products of the various metabolic processes are removed through the breath. A constant supply of fresh air for bedtime helps this process. An open window is of great benefit to aiding the body during sleep.

How one breathes during this sleep is extremely important. Left to its own devices, the body returns to slow, deep diaphragmatic breathing during sleep. The diaphragm slowly rises and falls, filling the body with life-sustaining oxygen. Unfortunately most of us tend to interfere with this natural process. Many people tend to sleep with their mouths wide open, a habit that often starts in childhood. Parents should be watchful of this and gently close the child's mouth whenever possible. Mouth breathing does not provide the deep respiration for the body that diaphragmatic breathing does.

When we sleep on our stomachs, the weight of the body prevents the diaphragm and the rib cage from properly expanding. Breathing in this position, we fill only the upper parts of the lungs. When we awaken we may feel as if we have not slept a wink. The best position for sleep is either on the back or on the side. Unfortunately very few of us sleep in either of these positions. As soon as we get into bed most of us automatically turn onto our stomachs and proceed to drift off to slumberland. So next time you crawl into bed get on your back or your side. Just as you relax and are beginning to fall asleep take notice of your breathing. The belly should be comfortably rising and falling as the chest also gently rises and falls with each unobstructed breath you take. Once you get used to this position you will probably find it preferable to sleeping on your stomach. Most likely you will awaken less tired and have a better supply of energy throughout the day because the body has had a chance to rid itself of accumulated waste gases as well as take in the benefits of vital oxygen. Should you awaken in the middle of the night, make sure that you check your position. If you have turned onto your stomach, immediately turn back over onto your side. In addition, when you awaken in the morning, check your position to see if you indeed did sleep on your side.

One of the most important keys to achieving a thorough night's rest is the ability to relax while going to sleep. If you let problems of the day intrude into your mind just before you retire, chances are your sleep will be uneven and usually disturbed with anxieties continually cropping up during the night. The time just before sleep should be one of the most pleasant periods of the entire day. Your mind should be filled with nothing but the most beautiful thoughts. Walks on the beach, standing in fields with nothing but the most beautiful wild flowers, being alone in a plane high above the city—all such mental images make for much more restful sleep than do thoughts of mergers, telephone calls or missed appointments.

Many people have forgotten how to fall asleep. Instead they attempt to force their body into rest through the use of sleeping pills. In fact, over two million Americans now put themselves to sleep chemically on a regular basis. Such behavior has become so ingrained in our social patterning that little thought is given to the effect of these drugs on our overall mental and physical functioning. Without even considering other methods of achieving a natural night's sleep, doctors seem to prescribe wantonly a whole range of sedatives to their patients, who then blindly swallow their routine tablet before bedtime. When you stop to think about it, you may realize that this is an utterly childish activity. Imagine an adult saying, "I can't sleep. I'm going to take this pretty pink pill and everything is going to be okay." It's all rather absurd. It just accentuates our lack of intelligent communication with our own bodies as well as a marked irresponsibility toward its needs and its care. Getting involved with tranquilizers or mood-altering tablets is a sultry affair. It's a silent addiction. This dependence begins in innocent and seemingly harmless ways. You might be at one of those points where everything is cracking all around you. What could be easier than a ten-minute visit to the doctor's office to get a month's supply of seemingly anxiety-free sleep? Suddenly you realize you have to have these pills in order to sleep. Being as lazy as we are and as habit-oriented as we are, such a pattern too easily becomes established, rapidly becoming the norm. On the part of both the doctor and the patient it seems that the issue of ingesting mood-altering drugs is both irresponsible and destructive.

For every beneficial response that the drugs provide there is an equally unpleasant and counterproductive result. Even though they relieve symptoms of anxiety relatively quickly, the serenity they produce is often followed by a more intense reoccurrence of the same tension and anxiety, which continues to build until once again relieved by a drug. These drugs by their very nature begin to alter the functioning of our nervous system. The sleep they create is a synthetic analogue of sleep, but not really restful sleep itself. By altering the biochemical activity of the brain, drugs begin to create an entirely new set of stimulus response situations within the body and the brain. These drugs function more like generalized Band-Aids covering a whole host of symptoms rather than remedying the cause. Similar and more effective results can be achieved through controlled breathing.

Ultimately the preference of doctors and sleep scientists

everywhere is to devise some method of sleep induction that is completely in accordance with the needs of the body, that is free from toxic side effects and is nonaddicting. Toward this end they have looked at everything from strenuous exercise and certain foods to warm milk. The most obvious answer is breathing.

It is quite possible to influence the central nervous system, to put our minds at ease and our bodies in a state of rest all through breathing. By increasing your oxygen intake before sleep, your body can ease itself away from the tensions of the day. Proper breathing throughout the night can assure a deep and restful sleep so that you wake up feeling refreshed and energetic rather than dopey and tired. Through controlled breathing you can increase the quality of rest you receive. You may even find that you need to sleep less.

The de-tense breath is extremely effective and useful on those evenings when your body is rigid with tension and your mind is speeding through a thousand different thoughts and problems. The de-tense breath releases all of the mental and physical tension in the body. Afterward you feel clean and empty of all stress and quickly drift off to sleep. The de-tense breath is best done after you have brushed your teeth, put on your night clothes and made all the preparations for bed. Unless you have an enormous bed, the de-tense breath is best done on the floor.

■ DE-TENSE BREATH

1. Lying flat on your back with your hands by your sides, close your eyes. Slowly begin to inhale the total breath through your nose. As you inhale, begin to raise your arms in an arc up and over your head.
2. Continue to inhale very slowly for the count of ten. As you reach ten, your arms should be at the floor and stretched out over your head. (Your elbows will be next to your ears.) See Fig. 17.
3. Hold the breath for ten counts.
4. As you exhale to a count of ten, slowly return your

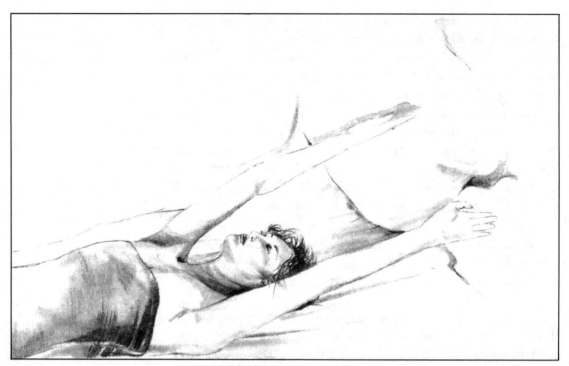

Fig. 17. De-tense Breath, Step 2. As you complete the inhalation, your arms should come to rest stretched over your head.

arms in the arc until they are resting alongside your body.

5. Repeat the exercise ten times.

6. Go to sleep.

With each inhalation you will begin to fall deeper and deeper into an almost dreamlike state. By lifting your arms up and over your head as you breathe you give your lungs the chance to expand fully and take in a larger supply of oxygen. This increased oxygen is invaluable for quieting nerves and producing a deep and restful sleep.

The de-tense breath not only solves difficulties of falling asleep but also prepares the body for a deeper and richer sleep. If at first you cannot fulfill the count of ten, breathe in five, hold five and release five. Then gradually work your way up to ten. As you raise your hands in the arc, feel as if the tips of your fingers are attached to puppet strings and are being pulled up and over your head. Just stretch slightly.

With each repetition you will feel your inhalations becoming deeper and more pleasant. As you raise your hands in the arc, feel as if you are pulling in the inhalation with your arms. And, in the exhalation as the hands return to the side, feel as if you are pushing out the exhalation. With each breath the interior of your head will feel as if the lights are growing dimmer and dimmer and your body is floating away. If you find yourself occasionally waking in the middle of the night after a few hours' sleep, the *return breath* will send you right back to sleep.

■ **RETURN BREATH**

1. Lying on your back in bed, close the right nostril with the right thumb.
2. Slowly inhale through the left nostril for ten counts. As you inhale, aim the breath for the spot in the center of your forehead.
3. Hold for ten counts.
4. Still holding the right nostril closed, exhale for ten counts.
5. Pause for five counts.
6. Close the left nostril with the middle finger.
7. Slowly inhale for ten counts, again aiming for that spot in the middle of the forehead.
8. Hold for a count of ten.
9. Still holding the left nostril closed, exhale for ten counts. Repeat the return breath ten times, after which you should quickly be on the way back to slumberland. When practicing the return breath watch your inhalations to make sure that they are silent. If they whistle at all, inhale at a slower, more even pace. The same thing applies to exhalations.

The *wave breath* is another exercise that is perfect for relaxing the body and mind before sleep.

■ **WAVE BREATH**

1. Lying on your back, inhale slowly through both nostrils in a steady but controlled stream.

2. As soon as you have inhaled the maximum amount of air possible without straining, immediately let the breath exhale by itself. Do not hold the breath or pause between inhalations.

3. When you have just finished exhaling, begin another inhalation, again without pausing.

4. Slowly repeat this exercise ten times.

5. Progressively take longer and longer with each inhalation and exhalation.

Another exercise for safely inducing sleep is the *pattern breath*.

■ PATTERN BREATH

In this breath the rhythm and pace of inhalation/exhalation is important.

1. Inhale slowly to the count of three.

2. Hold for six counts.

3. Exhale for the count of three. In the next breath add an extra count to the inhalation, retention and exhalation. With each new breath continue to add an extra count.

4. Inhale slowly for four counts.

5. Hold for seven counts.

6. Exhale at four counts. Add another count with the next breath cycle.

7. Inhale for five counts.

8. Hold for eight counts.

9. Exhale for five counts.

Continue the pattern breath until you reach an inhalation/exhalation count of ten. If at the end of the entire exercise you have not practically drifted off to sleep, repeat the entire exercise two more times.

Emptying the lungs of as much stale air as possible before you retire helps the body perform its natural cleaning process during sleep. The *snake breath* is a good exercise for refreshing the lungs before sleep.

■ SNAKE BREATH

1. Inhale the total breath.

2. Slowly exhale, making a hissing sound through the mouth. Keeping your teeth closed, exhale as if saying the letter "S." See Fig. 18.

3. Repeat ten times. Afterward you will feel pleasantly clean and tired.

Each of the exercises in the sleep program is designed to relax and aerate the body before sleep. They should be done slowly before bed. For many, the de-tense breath is the most effective; others may find the return breath or the wave breath more relaxing. Try them all and find which one provides you with the deepest and most restful sleep.

Fig. 18. Snake Breath, Step 2. Open your lips and push the breath out between closed teeth.

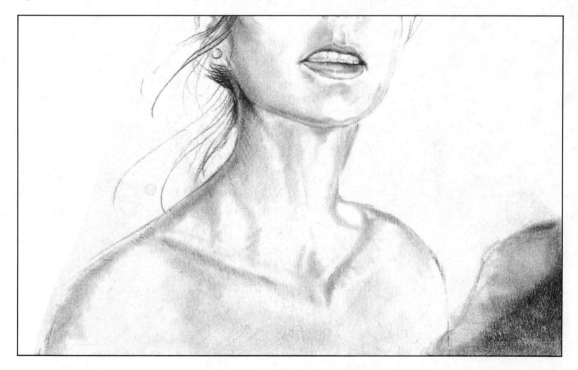

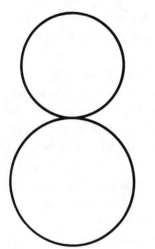

EXERCISE PROGRAM

DESPITE ALL THE BENEFITS and pleasures associated with exercise, people will still develop any excuse to avoid it. Either they are too tired, too old or have no time. Interestingly these three excuses often evolve precisely because of the lack of exercise. Exercise heightens our energy levels, slows down the aging process and helps us become more efficient. Somehow we have all been instilled with the erroneous notion that exercise is unrewarding, unrelentless work. We have failed to understand that there are different types of exercise as well as different qualities of exercise. Breathing happens to be one of them. In fact breathing is in many ways one of the most complete forms of exercise.

Breathing can expand the chest, strengthen and tone various muscles, stimulate and massage the internal organs and provide oxygen for the vital functioning of the entire body. When breathing is combined with specific movements it will affect the functioning of the nervous system, the cardiovascular system, the brain, the skin and the muscular system. Breathing exercises require no special equipment, clothes or space. They can be done anywhere, any time. Many of the breathing exercises in this chapter are also ideal for individuals confined to bed who wish to maintain their muscle tone and healthy circulation.

For some people, lifting weights is an extremely hazardous undertaking. The strain on the skeletal structure often proves to be too much, thus injuring joints and tendons. The following three exercises all work the muscles of the upper chest area without any of the potential strain incurred from weight lifting. They are perfect for staying in shape without tightening and stiffening the muscles. For some people muscles that are forged from weights do not always age well and often inhibit graceful movement.

During the work day we tend to let our chests collapse inward as we slump over our desks while attending to work. Not only does this seriously decrease our ability to have full inhalations, but the major muscles of the chest area begin to atrophy and lose their tone.

■ HORIZONTAL CHEST EXPANSION

1. Inhale the total breath.
2. Make a fist with both hands and extend the arms to shoulder level.
3. Forcefully swing the arms horizontally as far back as possible, then bring them all the way forward and swing them back again.
4. As the arms swing toward the back, exhale in a quick sniff about a quarter of the air in your lungs. Swing your arms to the front without inhaling and, as they swing back again, exhale another quarter. After four sniff exhalations, inhale a full breath as you bring the arms back to the front.

The rhythm is:

> Inhale
> Swing back, sniff out
> swing front

swing back, sniff out
swing front
swing back, sniff out
swing front
swing back, sniff out
swing front, inhale
swing back, sniff out
swing front
swing back, sniff out
swing front
swing back, sniff out
swing front
swing back, sniff out
swing front, inhale.

Repeat the exercise for a total of ten inhalations. The swing of the arms helps tone the deltoid and pectoral muscles of the chest and upper arms as well as stretch and expand the width of the chest cavity. By deeply inhaling and holding the breath your body then makes greater use of the oxygen during the workout.

■ VERTICAL CHEST EXPANSION

1. Inhale as you slowly lift your straightened arms out in front of you and up over your head. Hold for twenty counts.
2. Exhale and lower your arms for ten counts.
3. Repeat ten complete inhalations.

The *vertical chest expansion* should be done as slowly as possible, giving every muscle an opportunity to be well worked and thoroughly stretched. The greater pectoral muscles of the chest, the broadest muscle of the back, and the larger round as well as the external oblique which extends down the sides of the body are all toned and tightened in this exercise. Most importantly, with each inhalation the rib cage is stretched, giving the lungs good space to expand to their capacity. This exercise may also be done one arm at a time.

■ CHEST INFLATION

1. Deeply inhale the total breath.

2. Place your palms just above your breast with your elbows extended toward your back. See Fig. 19.

3. Holding the breath, pull the elbows as close to the body as possible, preferably touching it.

4. Hold for three seconds.

5. Release.

6. While holding the breath, continue to pull back and then release for ten counts.

7. Keeping the hands in place, fully exhale. Contract the diaphragm once or twice after the initial exhalation to push out residual air.

8. Repeat the entire exercise ten times.

The chest inflation stretches and works the muscles of the entire upper chest and also expands the rib cage to create increased area for lung expansion.

Being confined to bed is a nuisance for anyone but especially for the physically active. Whether it's a weekend of rest and recuperation or six weeks with a broken foot from jogging, serving time in bed can seriously affect your physical and mental agility. Through breathing it is possible to carry on a full regimen of exercises without in any way straining or interfering with your rate of recovery. In fact, by maintaining a level of physical fitness while confined to bed, chances are that you will recover quicker than if you were just to lie there. While in bed with an injury or an illness our intake of oxygen decreases greatly from what it usually is when we are up and about. Maintaining an exercise discipline while bedridden greatly improves our mood. With any period of bed restriction, we are undoubtedly bound to experience bouts of depression. All we ever think about is will we ever get well. During these times it is to our benefit if we divert our attention to something more constructive.

The *sea-breeze breath* utilizes both the diaphragm and the intercostals to fill the lungs to their maximum potential. Aside from exercising these muscles and expanding the entire chest and rib cage, the sea-breeze breath also provides

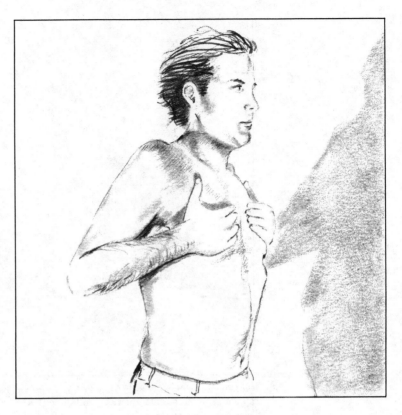

Fig. 19. Chest Inflation, Step 2. Pull your elbows in toward the spine to expand the upper chest.

stimulus to the imagination and refocuses the mind and the body away from the illness.

■ SEA-BREEZE BREATH

1. Lying on your back, tilt your head back so that it rests on the uppermost section of the skull. See Fig. 20.
2. Close your eyes and imagine that you are at the sea shore with beautiful sand, clear blue water, hovering sea gulls and radiant sun.
3. Now sniff in the total breath filled with imaginary sea air. As the inhalation approaches the chest, push the breast area as high into the air as it will go. This will also stretch the lower back while you finish the inhalation.
4. Hold this position and the inhalation for as long as is pleasantly possible.
5. As you watch the tides wash in, slowly exhale. During

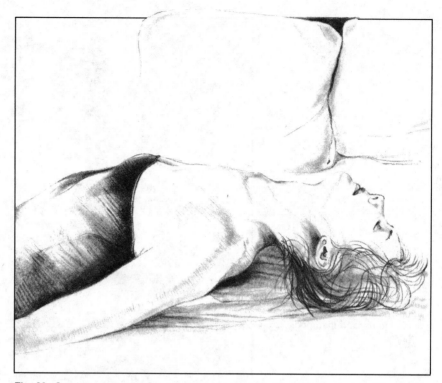

Fig. 20. Sea-breeze Breath, Step 1. Rest your head on the uppermost part of the skull to form a slight arch under the neck and upper back.

subsequent inhalations you may slowly turn your head from side to side just as if you were out for a nice tan, giving the neck area a stretch. Breathing as deeply as possible, let the aroma of fresh sea air fill your head. Continue the exercise for as long as you wish. For some it may take a bit of practice to get your imagination working. After a few breaths, it will come.

■ ARM-PRESS BREATH

1. Lie on your back with your arms at your side. Inhale through the nose a total breath.

2. Hold the breath. Push down with your palms into the bed or the floor as if you were doing a reverse push-up. Arch your back, raising your chest as high as possible. Feel the stretch from the chest down to the abdomen as

well as the exercising of the forearms and the biceps.
Hold for a count of ten.

3. Release the pressure of your palms and slowly let the
back slide back down onto the bed.

4. Exhale as you lower the body.

The arm-press breath fully inflates the lungs, stretches
the spine, as well as exercises the major muscles of the chest
and arms. It is not a strenuous exercise, yet it does produce
positive results in terms of maintaining muscle tone and
flexibility.

■ STOMACH PUMP

1. Lie on your back with your hands at your sides.

2. Each complete inhalation will be made up of ten short
sniffs of air. With each sniff of air push your belly as far
out as it will go, then sniff in a breath.

3. After each sniff, let the belly relax.

4. Continue the sniffing until you have sniffed in ten
times and filled your lungs with fresh air.

5. Relax and hold the air for five counts.

6. To exhale, reverse the inhalation process. Pull the
belly in quickly and sniff out. Again, allow ten sniffs for a
complete exhalation. The stomach pump concentrates on
working the full complement of abdominal muscles
without producing strain or exhaustion.

■ LEG PRESS

1. Lie on your back. Bring your knees up so that they are
close to your chin.

2. Place a hand on each knee cap. As you inhale a total
breath, pull down on both knees, bringing them as close
to the chest as possible.

3. By pulling the knees toward the chest you should be
able to raise your lower back off the bed.

4. Exhale and let the arms relax their pull on the knees.

5. Repeat ten times.

The leg press keeps the legs flexible. It also stimulates the base of the spine, which during extended periods of bed rest may become sore and make the entire body uncomfortable.

■ HELICOPTER BREATH

1. Lie on your left side. Bring your knees up slightly so that you are in a semifetal position.
2. Your right arm should be stretched out by your side.
3. Begin to inhale a total breath. As you do so bring your arm out in back of you and begin a circular motion around your body as if it were a helicopter blade.
4. As the arm begins to pass over the head you should begin the exhalation.
5. The arm should continue the circle and come to rest again on the side.
6. Repeat ten times. Then roll over on your right side and, using the left arm, repeat the exercise.

The helicopter breath provides a good stretch for the side muscles as well as a good stretch for the entire arm.

■ BAR-BELL BREATH

1. Lying on your back, inhale the total breath. Make a fist of each hand and raise them both so that they are straight up in the air.
2. As you exhale, lower each arm out to the side of the body, much like the motion of a windshield wiper. Do not let the fists touch the bed. Keep them about an inch off the bed and hold for ten counts.
3. Inhale and slowly bring the fists back up into the air over the body. Hold for ten seconds.
4. Exhale as you lower the hands and repeat the exercise ten times.

In this exercise you are creating your own bar bells, which will serve as sufficient weight to tone the muscles of the arms and chest. By holding your hands above the bed surface sufficient muscle tension occurs to strengthen the pectorals and biceps. The deep breathing enhanced by the movement of the arms further promotes the expansion and development of the chest.

■ PISTON BREATH

This is a wonderful breath that quickly tightens the stomach muscles, massages the liver and intestines, strengthens the diaphragm and stimulates the circulation.

1. Sitting cross-legged, inhale and exhale the total breath.
2. Forcefully contract the stomach to push out the last bit of residual air.
3. Let the stomach snap back out as you sniff in the inhalation.
4. Continue this in-and-out contraction and release of the abdomen as you breathe. The breath will sound like a choo-choo train.
5. Start out slowly but gradually increase the tempo of your breathing rate. Eventually you should have your breathing going at such a pace that you will almost sound "out of breath." Aside from exercising the entire abdomen and massaging the internal organs, the piston breath is quite good for creating body warmth for those who are habitually cold. The piston breath stimulates the circulation through the body, which is so necessary for those confined to bed.

■ RIB EXPANSION BREATH

1. Standing, place your hands on the side of your ribs just below your breasts.
2. Slowly inhale, starting with the abdomen, next filling the rib-cage area and then the upper chest. Pay special attention to the rib cage. When you fill it, slightly pull in the diaphragm and let the rib cage expand as far out to the side as possible. With your hands you will feel the ribs expanding laterally.

3. As you hold the breath with your hands still on the side, pull up on the rib cage and then gently "work" it by expanding and contracting the muscles out to the side. To do so you will have to lift the diaphragm slightly with each expansion.

4. Exhale about a quarter of the amount of air in your lungs, stop and again "work" the rib cage for five counts.

5. Continue to exhale and pause to work the ribs until you have completed the exhalation. After a few repetitions you will find that you have greater control over the entire rib cage. The strengthening of these muscles increases the area for lung expansion and corrects posture difficulties. Continued practicing of the rib expansion breath will do much to enhance your breathing.

■ BACK STRETCH

1. While standing, place your hands behind your back and clasp them together. They should be resting just below your lower back.

2. Fully inhale the total breath. Concentrate on inflating the upper chest area.

3. From your lower back, push your clasped hands out and away from the body as far as they will go. Then raise them as high as they will go. Hold for ten seconds. Make sure you keep the elbows straight.

4. Return the hands to their resting position.

5. Exhale.

The *back stretch* exercises those muscles around the shoulder area that often receive little attention. Tension often accumulates at the upper back and the tops of the shoulders before heading onto other parts of the body. By flexing the muscles you squeeze out the tension before it has an opportunity to create a headache or an ulcer. This exercise is also extremely useful for filling in those hollow areas just along the top of the shoulder. Aside from strengthening muscles of the upper back, the stretch also firms and works the major muscles of the upper arms and lower arms along the pectorals. In short, the back stretch breath is a true weight lifter's exercise but without the weights.

■ ARM STRETCH

1. Standing, extend your arms outward from the body to the sides and hold them at shoulder height.
2. Keeping your arms extended, slowly inhale the total breath.
3. Hold for ten counts.
4. Exhale.
5. Do not breathe for ten counts.
6. Keeping the arms extended from the body, repeat the same cycle of inhalation/exhalation five times.
7. After the fifth exhalation, bring the hands down to the sides.
8. Do two complete sets of five inhalations/exhalations.

The *sitting breath* stretches the spine, the leg muscles and the stomach area. If practiced regularly, it will give great flexibility to the entire body.

■ SITTING BREATH

1. Sit on the floor with your legs stretched out in front of you.
2. Take your left leg and bring it back under the body so that you are sitting on the heel.
3. Now close your eyes and inhale the total breath.
4. Hold for ten counts.
5. As you exhale, lean forward and grab your right foot. Your head should come to rest on your right knee. However, if you are not properly stretched out, this may take some time. Hold this position for twenty counts.
6. Release the foot and come back up to your original position.
7. Now, reverse the feet, stretching your left foot out in front of you and bringing your right foot in under the body, sitting on the right heel.

8. Inhale the total breath.

9. Hold for ten counts.

10. As you exhale, lean forward and grab your left foot. Your head should come to rest on your left knee. Hold for twenty counts.

11. Release the foot and come back up to your original position.

12. Continue this exercise for ten stretches on each leg.

The *seal breath* exercises and tightens the hips, buttocks and stomach area.

■ SEAL BREATH

1. Sit with your spine erect.

2. Close your eyes and inhale the total breath.

3. To seal in the breath, place your tongue on the roof of the mouth and swallow. As you swallow you will feel the throat tighten. Hold it closed, locking the throat.

4. As you hold the throat closed, squeeze the buttocks and the stomach first in and then up.

5. Hold for twenty counts.

6. Release the buttocks, stomach and throat muscles, then very slowly exhale the breath through the nose.

7. Inhale the total breath. Then, without holding, exhale the breath.

8. Slowly inhale the total breath and again repeat the locking of the throat and the squeezing of the stomach and the buttocks.

9. Repeat this exercise ten times.

The *contract breath* concentrates on tightening the stomach and chest muscles.

■ CONTRACT BREATH

1. Comfortably sit on the floor with your legs crossed and rest your hands on your knees.

2. Close your eyes and deeply inhale the total breath through the nose.

3. As you hold the breath for fifteen counts, press your chin into the chest and contract the stomach.

4. Lift the head, straighten the body and exhale through the nose for seven counts.

5. Keeping the lungs empty, again press the chin into the chest and contract the throat. Hold for fifteen counts.

6. Lift the head, straighten the body and inhale the total breath through the nose.

7. Slowly repeat the exercise five times.

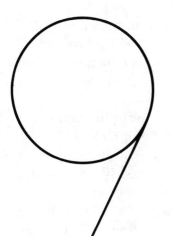

PREVENTION PROGRAM

LIKE ANY OTHER COMPLEX piece of machinery, the human body needs maintenance. This of course includes exercise, rest and nutrition. People often think of prevention as a lot of work, yet they wouldn't think twice about spending time and money to tune up their car. The key is to incorporate a preventive program into your daily activities so that it becomes second nature, to pursue life in such a way that you continually reap benefits rather than harm. In the prevention program we will look at various ways that breathing can be used to enhance our health and aid in the prevention of disease.

Toward actively preventing disease, it is important occasionally to monitor your breathing and note any irregularities. As illness approaches it quietly disrupts your normal respiration pattern. You may feel your air passages actually narrow with the onset of a cold. Breathing often becomes shallow, and exhalations usually make a slight whispering sound when any infectious disease is beginning to take hold. Just before the disease hits, it may seem as if you are hardly breathing at all. It is at these times when you probably feel the least like paying attention to your breathing. But if you notice the change in time and the breath is corrected, chances are quite good that you will avoid any illness at all. Once you have established a healthy breathing pattern, periodically check to make sure it is retained.

The main purpose of the lungs is to rid the body of waste gases that accumulate as the by-product of metabolic activity. As the cells perform their jobs they give off by-products just as in any industrial manufacturing process. If these wastes are not removed through the body's main excretory organs such as the lungs, skin or stomach they begin to build up. They then recirculate throughout the body, acting as "gunk" that clogs up the machinery.

Many of the respiratory problems that affect our chest and lungs and eventually our entire body can be prevented through proper breathing. As stale air accumulates in the lungs from insufficient exhalations, this dead air becomes a breeding ground for germs and disease. With full ventilation of the lungs we can quickly cut down on the amount of colds and bronchial complications we encounter every year, especially in winter.

The common cold is probably one of the most widespread ailments in the world, but after all these years there is very little that has been discovered that relieves us of its symptoms, much less prevents it entirely. A great deal can be done through proper breathing to ward off the onslaught of winter colds.

During the colder times of the year we exercise much less, so our lungs are not given the opportunity to ventilate the body properly. In addition we are usually breathing stale dry air which is often germ-prone. The windows are closed and the heat is on. Continually breathing this dry air tends to interfere with the natural defense mechanism of the respiratory system. Remember, the lungs like warm, moist air.

To complicate the problem of winter breathing, we often expose our respiratory tract from one extreme of air to another. Outdoors the air is cool, while indoors it is hot. It is no wonder that we have such respiratory problems during the winter. These vast differences in air temperature make it especially important to breathe through the nose. In this way you will insure that the lungs are being fed moist warm air that is as clean and germ-free as possible. We should slow down our breathing rate as well. Take the air in through the nose at a slow, steady rate, giving it sufficient time to be moistened and warmed. You should also make sure that you increase your intake of fluids so that the body will maintain a proper moisture balance, which is especially important in the nasal passage and down the trachea.

By emphasizing exhalation, you will rid the body of as much dead air as possible. This will dramatically reduce your chances of catching cold. Try to keep a window open just a crack to allow in fresh air. Investing in a humidifier will also greatly decrease your respiratory complications during the winter. Probably more than any other factor affecting our winter health, preventive breathing can do much to alleviate the traditional winter cold.

Because breathing plays such a crucial role in our winter health, its interference by a nasty cold will only increase our miseries. Our nasal passages become blocked. Our chest is often congested and we find ourselves wheezing instead of breathing. The suffering seems as if it will last forever. Again, an ounce of prevention is worth a pound of cure.

One of the first signs of an approaching cold is the feeling of chilliness throughout the body. If you have begun to feel chilly, you may wish to check your breathing. It is probably slow and shallow, making a whispering noise with each exhalation. The first step in preventing this oncoming cold is to thoroughly clean out the lungs of stale air and to warm the body at the same time. These can both be accomplished through the *hissing breath.*

■ HISSING BREATH

1. Inhale the total breath.
2. Hold for three counts.
3. Part your lips and teeth ever so slightly. By

contracting your stomach and chest muscles, strongly exhale in a strong "hissss."
4. Immediately following the hissing exhalation, inhale a total breath and again exhale by hissing.
5. Repeat ten times.

One of the most uncomfortable symptoms of a cold or any of the other respiratory complications is the inability to breathe. Aside from being tired, most of our discomfort comes from chest congestion. Coughing is our natural mechanism for breaking up and releasing this excess accumulation of mucous from the chest. When we have an excess of mucous we either have a first-rate infection and the body is pouring out mucous in an attempt to flush the disease out of the system or our defenses are so weak that the mucous system is overstimulated. Sometimes the mucous is so thick that we must cough away for hours without even making a dent in the accumulation. Meanwhile, our breathing becomes even more confined and limited to the upper chest. Of course, one of the first things we want to do is reinstate our breathing, getting as much air into the lungs as possible while at the same time breaking up the congestion.

Percussion therapy is used in many hospitals to help patients who are overwhelmed with chest congestion. With the following *chest percussion breath* you can help loosen up a great deal of mucous accumulations in the chest area and hasten the passing of the cold.

■ **CHEST PERCUSSION BREATH**

1. Inhale the total breath.
2. Hold for fifteen counts.
3. Point your elbows toward the back of the body with your fists resting at the sides of your ribs. While you retain the breath, lightly pound the sides of your ribs, moving from top to bottom and back again.
4. Exhale.
5. Repeat this light pounding over the chest area.
6. Exhale and repeat. This exercise helps loosen accumulated mucous that often gets into the out-of-the-way places in the lungs.

Once an illness strikes it can be further complicated by the appearance of a fever. Although a fever can leave us feeling on the verge of death, it is actually a blessing in disguise. It is the body's own method of burning up the toxic wastes that created the disease in the first place. During the fever the body is generating an internal chemical fire to sterilize its own environment. Often the best treatment for the disease *and* the fever is just to let the fever burn itself out. The *fever breath* will do a great deal to relieve your discomfort and assist the body in cleaning house.

■ FEVER BREATH

1. Roll back your tongue, placing the tip on the roof of the mouth. Spread your lips in a grin and suck in a total breath.
2. Open your mouth as wide as possible and exhale in one long "haaaw." Start the exhalation from the very bottom of your stomach and let it continue up into the mid-area and finally the upper chest.

One of the most annoying aspects of any cold is the sinus headache and the constant running nose that make you feel as if you are swimming under water. Both of these symptoms are a result of the body working to rid itself of accumulated toxic matter. Swallowing antihistamines and squirting nose sprays sometimes relieves the symptoms of the cold but not the cold itself. These drugs appear to end the cold merely by shutting down the body's own natural defense reaction. However, this does not solve the problem. People who rely on chemical agents to quiet down the cold seem to experience frequent colds with increasing severity exactly because they have not gotten to the root of the problem, which may require a change in diet or a period of rest or exercise.

In the early twentieth century at health spas throughout northern Europe people with respiratory problems were cured through various inhalation therapies. Large steam rooms were created where patients inhaled the beneficial vapors of various herbs such as mints and eucalyptus. These herbs loosened the accumulated mucous of the bronchial tubes and the upper lungs.

There are various inhalation therapies that can be performed at home. They will allow the body to drain the congestion and the mucous without resorting to drugs. By using these therapies you can help the body rid itself of the accumulations of germs and dust that are trapped in the mucous. These inhalations gently dislodge and loosen the mucous, eventually cleaning out the entire bronchial system. And as is the nature with prevention, you do not have to wait until you are miserably sick, gasping for air. It is a good idea to do a mild eucalyptus inhalation for a few minutes once a week just to keep the bronchial area clean, especially with the dust and particulate matter we breathe these days. The inhalations are also especially beneficial during the winter for helping the nasal passageways stay warm and moist.

In performing the following two inhalations you will find that after about ten minutes a great deal of mucous will start to flow either from your nose and/or your throat. By all means pause to blow your nose to make yourself more comfortable. If the cold and the congestion are very severe and breathing is extremely difficult, repeat the steaming several times during the day until the passageways are clear from congestion.

■ EUCALPYTUS INHALATION

1. Bring a two-quart pot of water to a rapid boil.
2. Add three tablespoons of eucalyptus tea or eucalyptus extract, cover and let steep for two minutes. (You can buy eucalyptus tea at a health-food store, the extract at a drugstore.)
3. Draping a large bath towel over your head, forming an "oxygen tent," remove the pot's cover and lean over the pot. Try to keep as much steam in as possible with the towel. Be careful not to burn yourself. If the steam is too hot, lift up the edges of the towel and let some escape.
4. Slowly breathe in through your mouth and out your nose. Then alternate, breathing in through your nose and

out your mouth. Continue this procedure for as long as the steam stays hot and effective. Whenever you feel you must expectorate or blow your nose, cover the pot and do so. If you must steam again, it is best to heat up a fresh pot of water and some fresh eucalpytus. Rest about an hour between steamings.

■ CIDER VINEGAR INHALATION

1. Heat to boiling in a large pot a half cup of apple cider vinegar and two cups of water. If you find this mixture too strong, add another cup of water but do try to keep it as strong as possible.
2. Draping a large bath towel over your head, forming an "oxygen tent," remove the pot's cover and lean over the pot. Try to keep as much steam in as possible with the towel. Be careful not to burn yourself. If the steam is too hot, lift the edges of the towel up and let some escape.
3. Slowly breathe in through your mouth and out your nose. Then alternate, breathing in through your nose and out your mouth. Continue this procedure for as long as the steam stays hot and effective. Whenever you feel you must expectorate or blow your nose, cover the pot to keep the steam in and do so. If you must steam again, it is best to heat up a fresh pot of water with a fresh batch of apple cider vinegar. Rest about an hour between steamings. This mixture is far more powerful than the eucalyptus. The cider vinegar drains and then dries up the mucous, whereas the eucalyptus just eases it out. Depending on the severity of your cold, choose whichever one you feel is most suitable.

One of the most common causes of headaches is the accumulation of tension in the neck which restricts the flow of blood to the head. In order to keep the neck flexible, we want to loosen the neck muscles to facilitate a good flow of oxygen. The *neck roll* is the perfect exercise to insure adequate oxygenation along with a relaxed neck, thus reducing the incidence of headaches.

■ NECK ROLL

1. Exhale and let your chin drop to your chest.
2. As you start to inhale the total breath, begin slowly to roll your head to the left. The inhalation should finish just as the back of the head comes to rest over the center of the spine. When you roll the head, let its own weight guide the rolling action.
3. As the head begins to roll to the right, start the exhalation. When you finish the exhalation and the roll, your chin should come to rest in the center of your chest.
4. Even though you are inhaling and exhaling, the exercise should be smoothly performed in one single roll. Perform the neck roll to the left five times, then switch direction and roll to the right five times.

If you have accumulated a lot of neck tension, you may hear a sound like grinding gravel as you roll your head. Eventually as you improve the circulation to this area, the sounds will disappear. Also during the roll you may feel a pulling of certain muscles in your shoulders and back. These too will loosen up and smooth themselves out with continued exercise. Coordination of the breathing with the rolling motion is extremely important in loosening up the musculature as well as improving the oxygen supply to the brain.

Along with breathing, the digestive process provides the body with its life-sustaining fuel. Often this process is interfered with due to tension, poor eating habits, or improper breathing. With our digestion not up to par, we may not be deriving all of the important energy available from the food we eat. This can weaken our vitality and our resistance. Oftentimes our stomachs need stimulation in order to aid the digestive process or to prevent blockages in the flow of food. Deep regular breathing does much to keep the natural peristaltic action of the stomach in shape. At times it is useful to aid the stomach through colonic massage in combination with breathing. By gently massaging the intestinal area, we insure a good supply of blood and oxygen to the stomach to aid digestion. We will also be providing a stimulating influence on the liver as well. These exercises should always be done on an empty stomach. Internal massage helps alleviate the build-up of toxic wastes from the organs that often leads to disease.

■ INTESTINAL MASSAGE I

1. Inhale the total breath and hold for ten counts. Then completely exhale.
2. Place your fingertips on the soft spot just under the place where the ribs first join together. Your palms will be resting on your ribs.
3. With your fingertips gently push the stomach area in about an inch. Let the stomach bounce back. Slide your hands down the ribs a notch and repeat. With each pressing in let the fingers do a little circular finger massage as well. Once you reach the waist level, work your way back up to the starting point. See Fig. 21.
4. Inhale the total breath. Exhale.
5. Repeat three times.

■ INTESTINAL MASSAGE II

1. Inhale the total breath. Hold for ten counts. Completely exhale.
2. Place your hands, one on top of the other, on your stomach just below the navel.
3. Pressing slightly with the heel of your hand, move in a circular motion and massage the stomach area. Continue to move outward in larger circles as if making a spiral. Once you have reached the outer limits of the stomach, reverse the process and work your way back in.
4. Slowly inhale the total breath.
5. Hold for twenty counts.
6. Slowly exhale for twenty counts.
7. Repeat the entire process three times.

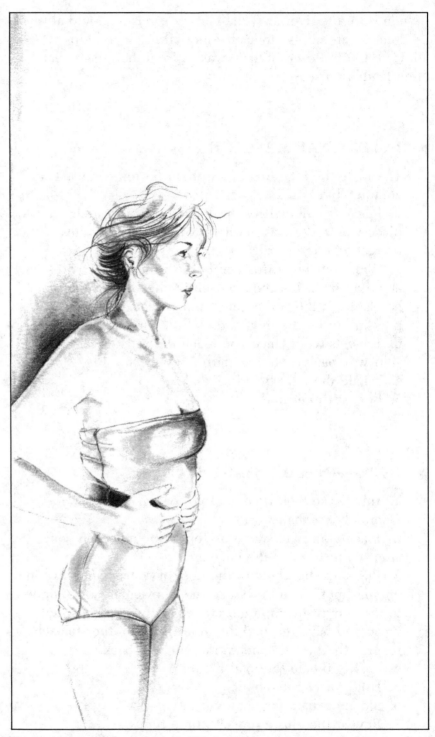

Fig. 21. Intestinal Massage I, Step 3. With the tips of your fingers, gently push in and massage the stomach.

■ KIDNEY MASSAGE

1. Standing erect, inhale the total breath.
2. Place the palms of your hands on the kidneys, which are located on the lower back just below the rib cage.
3. Lean forward from the waist so that your trunk is parallel to the floor. Then exhale.
4. Inhale a total breath.
5. Now, to exhale very gently press down on the kidneys with the balls of your palms to push out the breath. It should take five pushes on the kidney to create complete exhalation.
6. Remain bent over. Inhale and again push the exhalation out with the palms of the hands.
7. Repeat three times.

Since so many disease problems first start because of improper digestion, it is important to keep the stomach in tone. We can stimulate its digestive properties through the *abdominal breath*. Aside from toning up the stomach itself, this breath naturally stimulates important peristaltic action throughout the intestines. This exercise provides a churning action for the gastric juices in the stomach and provides the overall area with beneficial stimulation. Use the abdominal breath to help alleviate constipation as well.

■ ABDOMINAL BREATH

1. Sit comfortably in a chair or on the floor. Your hands should be resting on your upper thighs.
2. Inhale the total breath.
3. Exhale completely by contracting the diaphragm and intestinal muscles as far in as possible in two stages. First pull in the stomach to exhale the majority of the air. With an additional quick contraction pull the stomach muscles as far back as possible to finish the exhalation.
4. Release the stomach and let the air naturally flow into the lower lungs around the stomach area, then the mid-range around the ribs and finally the upper chest.
5. Repeat the two-step exhalation process.

6. Continue the exercise so that you are inhaling and exhaling at a somewhat rapid rate.

This two-step exhalation is best done between meals. It strengthens and massages the internal abdominal muscles and facilitates digestion and elimination. It should be practiced at least once a day.

Any change in altitude or pressure can drastically alter our breathing pattern. The very process of respiration depends on a delicate balance of various atmospheric pressures both inside and outside of the lungs. Pressure changes incurred as we gain altitude can cause discomfort throughout the body. Earaches, nausea and even heart strain can all be brought on by more rarefied air and higher altitudes. Since not many of us climb the Andes every day, our most common experience with change in pressure and altitude is the airplane flight. Despite the comfort of modern jets, there are many people who are still quite sensitive to being up high in the air. Take-off, landing and turbulence are usually these people's weak spots. The symptoms of nausea, headache and earache are often brought on by the change in the quantity and quality of oxygen. By altering your breathing pattern to compensate for the changes in pressure and altitude you can alleviate much of the physical discomfort that often accompanies flying.

The *take-off breath* will help open the ears and prevent that feeling of thickheadedness during the flight. By regularly oxygenating the body while in the air you can overcome any of the sensitivities you may experience during flying. It is a simple breath that should be done slowly during sudden changes in altitude and of course with each take-off and landing.

■ TAKE-OFF BREATH

1. Tilt your head back slightly. Open your mouth and yawn while inhaling. Take in as much air as possible.
2. Exhale through the mouth and swallow.
3. Repeat as often as necessary.

Experiencing turbulence in a plane creates a certain emotional anxiety in every passenger, not to mention the discomfort one feels in the pit of the stomach as the plane is tossed around. At this point your body is really being put through the pressurized mill. The *turbulence breath* is a way to calm your nerves, steady the body and gently increase the level of oxygen in the blood. The purpose of the visualization in the exercise is to focus the mind away from the physical discomfort and the possible tension that the passenger might be experiencing. This exercise will help maintain the body until equilibrium is reached. It should be performed slowly and with just a thin, steady stream of air entering or leaving the nostrils.

■ TURBULENCE BREATH

1. Lean back in your chair, close your eyes and tilt your head slightly backward.
2. Very slowly, inhale the total breath, only this time do not inflate your stomach as much as you usually do. The breath should be inhaled to a count of ten. It often helps with the discomfort and with the breathing itself to visualize yourself climbing ten stairs.
3. As soon as you have fully inhaled, begin the descent down the stairs with an exhalation of ten counts.
4. Continue the breath during the turbulence.

Although most of today's seagoing vessels are engineered to avoid severe rocking motion that can cause sea sickness, it does still happen. Needless to say, if you have a sensitive stomach, eat lightly or don't eat at all. As soon as the first signs of queasiness appear, begin the *sea breath,* which concentrates on the exhalations. By pressing your tongue to the roof of the mouth you will help quiet your active stomach.

■ SEA BREATH

1. Standing or sitting, tilt your head back and inhale the total breath but only so your lungs are about three quarters full.

2. As you hold the breath, press your tongue tightly against the roof of your mouth. Hold the breath for seven counts.

3. Looking slightly downward, vigorously exhale half of the breath, pause and exhale again. Be sure to get all the air out of the lungs without straining.

4. Repeat as necessary.

Apparently, hiccups have no preventive function in the body but instead are a symptom of excitement of specific nerve endings in the digestive system. A favored remedy has always been to hold the breath. Usually the nerves are so excited that holding the breath becomes an impossibility. A better yet similar solution is the *hiccup breath.*

■ HICCUP BREATH

1. Inhale a short total breath, about three seconds in duration.

2. Place the tongue against the roof of the mouth with mild pressure. Hold for seven seconds.

3. Exhale. Before you inhale, place the tongue against the roof of the mouth with mild pressure and hold for seven seconds.

4. Return to step #1. After three or four complete repetitions the hiccups should disappear.

■ PAIN

Pain is an extremely personal sensation. Words can never express to another person the crippling discomfort you may be feeling. Each person varies in his or her reaction to pain. No matter how much we dislike pain, it is primarily a protective mechanism. It is pain that lets us know when we are about to burn our hand on the stove or rip our skin to shreds on a barbed-wire fence.

Reactions to pain differ from person to person and time to time. A visit to the dentist may cause one person to faint, while another may have half his mouth drilled away without

Novocain and without wincing. The chemistry of pain is terribly complex, involving the stimulation of certain centers of the brain that interact with nerves in the skin and other tissues.

The following pain program is of enormous use both in everyday conditions and in emergencies involving pain. A good deal of the pain is due to the surprise of its attack and the fear of serious repercussions. Knowing that you are able to handle a great many painful sensations by yourself will help you reassert your sense of control and enhance your tolerance for pain. You become less afraid of pain, knowing that you are quite capable of controlling and rechanneling that energy. Like anything, pain becomes more manageable once the attention it has worked so hard to gather is focused into other areas.

Pain is, in part, dependent on certain muscular and mental tension for its existence. If we can just relax our bodies the pain diminishes remarkably. The most important factor in using any breath to alleviate painful sensations is to remember to change our breathing the second that the pain hits. When pain strikes it is accompanied by irregular breathing patterns. If we control our breathing as soon as pain appears, this not only alleviates much of the pain but also frees the mind from fear and tension, allowing it to cope with any immediate emergency that might be at hand. We cannot afford to allow pain to cripple our alertness, especially when clear thinking is required to remove ourselves from immediate danger.

The following exercises will do a great deal toward managing pain. Be sure to put all your concentration on the exhalations and not on the pain.

■ STOP-PAIN BREATH

1. Inhale a total breath as soon as you feel pain.
2. Without pausing, immediately exhale forcefully through the nostrils as if you were a bull getting ready to attack. Throughout the exercise the emphasis should be on strong forceful exhalations that are longer in length

than the inhalations. Your diaphragm plays a vital role in this exercise. The exhalations are literally *pushed* out by quickly contracting the diaphragm. Let the diaphragm collapse as far into the stomach as possible until it can't possibly push back any further. Then with the onrushing new inhalation let it recoil as you take in as much air as you can hold.

3. Continue to breathe in and out with great force, literally pushing the pain out of the body. Gradually begin to slow down the rhythm, taking longer and deeper inhalations as the pain diminishes.

At one time or another we all get some sort of injection, either a shot of Novocain at the dentist's or when we have blood samples taken. Although the pain is momentary it is nonetheless unpleasant. The *wind breath* can be used whenever we anticipate physical discomfort; it may also be used interchangeably with the stop-pain breath. Next time you get an injection at the doctor's office do three or four repetitions of the wind breath before the injection. Ask the nurse or doctor to insert the needle as you begin your third exhalation. Your pain will be greatly minimized. As the injection is being given, continue the breath.

■ WIND BREATH

1. Inhale deeply the total breath as if taking in one long sniff of air.

2. To exhale, slightly part the lips and force the air out of the opening, as if you were trying to whistle. The exhalations should be long and strong, as if you were blowing the pain out of the body.

3. Continue breathing with long exhalations until the pain subsides.

There are many times when we simply do not feel well, yet we can't seem to locate the cause or nature of our illness. Maybe we feel tired or a cold is coming on, or maybe our body just aches. It may be we are on our way to a major breakdown of all physical systems, or we may be under extreme mental stress. In this instance rushing off to a doctor when the symptoms are so vague is not always the best decision, especially if you are unable to describe the complaint. Sometimes the best treatment for such free-floating symptoms is to lie down, relax and just breathe. Often the symptoms will disappear or you will become clear enough and in touch enough with your body to locate exactly what is bothering you.

During the exercise try not to structure the breath pattern at all; just let yourself breathe. The only requirement is that you inhale and exhale deeply. Do not focus on whatever is bothering you or your worries of the day. This is recess. Your only job is to lie down and breathe.

■ JUST BREATHING

1. Lie on your back on the floor in a quiet room. Close your eyes.
2. Place your arms in their most comfortable position, either at your side, outstretched or clasped behind your head.
3. Slowly inhale the total breath.
4. Exhale.
5. You need not follow any specific pattern of breathing. Just breathe in the most comfortable fashion for as long as you feel like it. Just relax.

10 PROLONGEVITY PROGRAM

SINCE THE BEGINNING of recorded history we have been looking for ways to extend out lives in terms of quality and number of years. A variety of elixirs, mechanical methods, diets and potions are continually created in an attempt to make us live longer, look more beautiful and be happier. Every culture has made its contribution to this never-ending and all-consuming search. From Egyptian embalming and Ponce de León's fountain of youth to royal jelly and cryogenics, we seem to pursue this goal with increasing voracity.

Recently medical science has begun to look seriously at and isolate the factors that cause aging. Scientists are attacking the subject from every possible angle in an effort to understand and eventually influence the aging process. Diet, stress, genetic patterning and environmental factors are all being considered in the search to conquer aging. The research is endless and fascinating.

But underlying everything is the basic goal to improve and extend the operation of our vital functions. That is, keep the heart pumping, the brain working, the blood moving and the lungs breathing. Of course, every aspect of the body is completely dependent on the respiration process and the oxygen it delivers to the body. It is a well-known fact that as we age our lungs begin to lose their elasticity, thus weakening their potential. As our breathing capacity begins to diminish, so too does the amount and quality of oxygen that is delivered to our cells, tissues and organs. Thus begins a rather vicious cycle of physical and mental decline. Feeling tired and old is the least of the complications brought on by reduced oxygen supply. Our brain, which is critically dependent on oxygen, along with our heart, begins to operate at less than optimum levels as our lungs take in less and less vital oxygen. It is here that a whole host of degenerative conditions have their inception. The key, then, for continued optimum living appears to be maintenance of the body not only through proper nutrition and exercises but more so through correct breathing. In this way, the body is supplied with maximum oxygen for overcoming many of the aging factors attributed to the decline of oxygen intake in later years.

The goal of the prolongevity program is to increase the capacity of our lungs to provide the body with life-sustaining oxygen. Through exercises we will focus on the health and functioning of our most important organs throughout the body. We will also learn various breathing rhythms that will enable us more fully to utilize each breath while reducing mental and physical stress that so often contributes to aging.

There is a critical interdependence between breathing and body function. As the heart is dependent on a continual oxygen supply, so too is the body dependent on the heart to create the circulating or delivering force for that oxygen supply. If the heart fails because of lack of oxygen, then the rest of the body is also denied oxygen. In certain cases of heart disease, the lack of oxygen occurs through physical obstruction of the blood in the carrying conduits. Both ventilation and the promotion of dependable oxygen supplies would appear to be of immense benefit in preventing heart failure or rebuilding the individual's strength after a heart attack.

Part of the program to enhance our lungs' ability to capture important oxygen from the air is to clean both the nasal passages and the lungs themselves from accumulating stale air. The *pressurized breath* stimulates the resilient action of the lungs, along with providing a powerful expulsion of dormant air.

■ PRESSURIZED BREATH

1. In one swift inhalation, breathe in the total breath.
2. With your thumb and second finger, clamp both nostrils shut and hold for a count of seven.
3. Now, still holding the nose closed, puff out your cheeks and fill them with as much air as possible without letting any slip out between the lips. Now pressurize this air by squeezing out the cheeks as far as they will go while simultaneously contracting the chest slightly. Hold for three counts. See Fig. 22.
4. Release the nose and vigorously exhale all at once through both the nose and the mouth.
5. Repeat five times.

Another method of stimulating and cleaning the lungs is the *one-sided breath,* which gives each side of the nasal passage and lungs a thorough cleaning.

■ ONE-SIDED BREATH

1. With your thumb close the right nostril. Now suck in a complete inhalation of the total breath through your left nostril.
2. Hold for three counts.
3. Exhale in one forceful stream from the left nostril.
4. Repeat three times, all the while keeping the right nostril closed.
5. Next, release your thumb and with your third finger close the left nostril.
6. Suck in a complete inhalation of the total breath through your right nostril.
7. Hold for three counts.

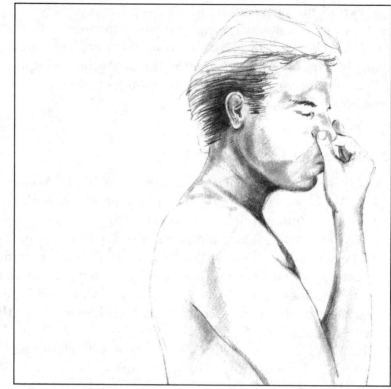

Fig. 22. Pressurized Breath, Step 3. Holding the nose closed, puff out the cheeks, fill with air and contract the chest.

8. Exhale in one forceful stream from the right nostril.
9. Repeat three times, all the while keeping the left nostril closed.

Most of us who have never breathed properly function with only a minimal level of satisfactory oxygen in our bloodstreams. This of course can slow down all of our thinking and metabolic processes. Without adequate oxygen our blood can become sluggish and thick with impurities, which can contribute to the aging process. The *super oxygen breath* can stimulate the inflow of oxygen into the body and aid in providing the purifying action of oxygen in the blood.

■ SUPER OXYGEN BREATH

1. Form your lips into the tiniest "O" possible, as if you were drinking iced tea from a straw.

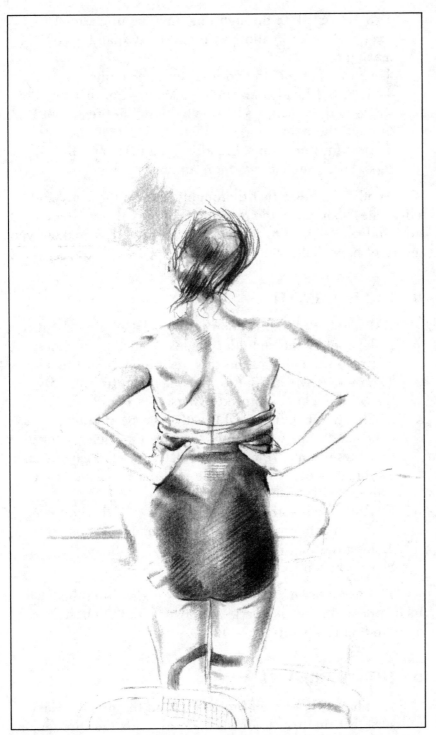

Fig. 23. Full Breath, Step 1. To help the lungs expand, place the thumbs on the spine pointing upward.

2. Slowly suck in through this tiny opening a total breath. Be sure to allow your chest to expand to its maximum.

3. Close your mouth and hold for five counts.

4. Tilt your head back slightly. Again form that tiny "O" shape with your lips and slowly blow the breath out through the hole.

5. Rest for ten counts, breathing regularly and then repeat the exercise two more times.

Another exercise that thoroughly aerates the body and eliminates stale air is the *full breath.* You will feel the chest area and ribs expand to their maximum potential, making you aware of how shallow your breath has been.

■ FULL BREATH

1. Place both thumbs pointing up on the spine about two inches below the shoulder blades. Your fingers should be resting on the side of the ribs just below breast level. The elbows will be out to the sides, pointing slightly to the back, looking a bit like wings. See Fig. 23.

2. Slowly inhale the total breath. The positioning of the hands and arms will greatly increase the capacity for the lungs to expand. You will especially feel the expansion as the breath begins to enter the mid-region of the chest. The ribs will lift up and out.

3. Hold the breath for twenty counts. Let the body get used to maximum expansion and proper aeration.

4. Keeping the hands in place, slowly exhale.

5. Repeat ten times.

The *horse breath* also helps to rid toxins from the bloodstream and gives gentle stimulation to the chest area surrounding the heart.

■ HORSE BREATH

1. Inhale a brief total breath through the mouth. Make sure that the breath touches and expands the three main areas of the lower stomach, rib cage and upper chest.

2. To exhale, relax your lips and let the breath rapidly flap the lips as if you were a horse.

3. Repeat three times.

As with the other breath exercises in this program, the *vigorous exhalation* helps clear the lungs of unwanted air while reducing and relieving stress from the body.

■ VIGOROUS EXHALATION

1. Standing straight with your legs eighteen inches apart, bend your knees slightly, as if you were riding a horse. Lower your buttocks a bit and lean forward so that your hands come to rest naturally on your legs about an inch above the knees. This position will be something of a standing squat.

2. Inhale a total breath through the nose.

3. Hold for two seconds.

4. Let the breath exhale itself through the open mouth. As soon as the exhalation is finished, squeeze in the abdomen three more times to push out the remaining air. You may make a huffing sound during these last three exhalations.

5. Close the mouth and do not inhale for the next four seconds.

6. Repeat the entire procedure three times. Then rest, stretch your legs and repeat the entire exercise three more times.

According to certain Eastern philosophies you are born into this world with a certain number of breaths rather than years to your lifetime. Your life ends not because of old age but because you have used up your breath quota. In the search for longevity methods were devised to slow down the breathing process, to utilize fully each breath to its fullest advantage and thereby to breathe less. If indeed this approach is correct, there are a few exercises that will enable us to enhance our lung volume, get more oxygen from each breath and thereby breathe slower. This approach of breathing more fully yet less often is not without its logic. Frequent or rapid breathing is often a sign of anxiety and tension, certainly a well-known killer in our day and age, whereas slower, deeper breathing allows the body to absorb larger amounts of oxygen, providing the cells with additional stimulus for activity and generation.

Slowing down the breath is a gradual process that requires the expansion of our lung capacity along with the alteration of our breathing rhythms. Over time, the body will accustom itself to breathing at a much slower rate while making more efficient use of the oxygen taken in.

■ SLOWING THE BREATH

1. Slowly inhale and exhale the total breath.
2. With your right thumb, close your right nostril. Now, slowly inhale the total breath through the left nostril for a count of ten.
3. With your fourth finger, close the left nostril and hold the breath for a count of twenty.
4. Keeping the left nostril closed, release the thumb and slowly exhale through the right nostril for ten counts. See Fig. 24.
5. Do not breathe for five counts.
6. Reverse the inhalation to the right nostril by closing the left nostril with the fourth finger. Inhale the total breath for ten counts.
7. Close the right nostril with the thumb and hold for twenty counts.
8. Keeping your right nostril closed, release your fourth finger and exhale slowly through the left nostril for ten counts.
9. Do not breathe for five counts. Repeat the above four times.
10. For the next round of slowing the breath, add five counts to every inhalation, retention and exhalation. Then repeat four more times. This completes one session of slowing the breath.
11. Each time you practice this exercise increase the inhalation, retention and exhalation for five counts. Once you have reached a maximum count of forty for the

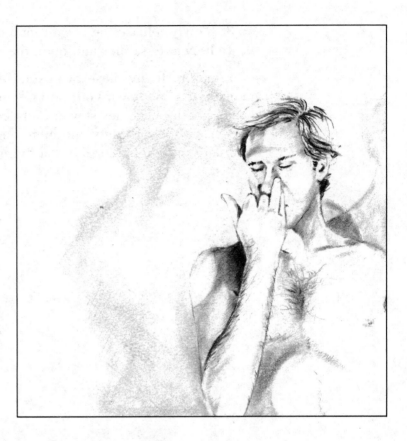

Fig. 24. Slowing the Breath, Step 4. Keeping the left nostril closed, release the thumb and exhale through the right nostril.

inhalation and exhalation you need not keep increasing the count unless you feel you are able to. Maintain this count each time you perform slowing the breath.

Another version of slowing the breath that offers a moment of quiet while regulating the breathing pattern is *slowing the breath II.*

■ **SLOWING THE BREATH II**

1. Close your eyes and sit comfortably in a chair. Focus both eyes on the tip of your nose. Inhale the total breath slowly through the nose for a count of ten.

2. As you hold the breath for a count of twenty, relax the shoulders and upper chest area, allowing the breath to seek its natural boundaries.

3. Slowly release the breath for a count of ten.
4. Repeat ten times and open the eyes.

From practicing these two exercises you should begin gradually to slow down your normal breathing process. As your breathing becomes slower and deeper you will find yourself with less anxiety and more energy—two very important ingredients for living a fuller life.

STRESS
AND EMOTIONS
PROGRAM

OUR RHYTHM OF BREATH accurately reflects our state of mind. For example, when we are absorbed in concentration, our breathing becomes deep and regular. If we are nervous, the breath then becomes shallow and irregular. Fear creates quick random gulps of air, while comfort is accompanied by steady and relaxed breathing.

Throughout the day we have a variety of breathing patterns that change along with our thoughts. Quite often people's inner states are reflected in their breathing. Next time you meet someone, listen to and watch how they breathe. Is their breathing slow and steady or quick and shallow? Is it noisy? Do they make a whistling noise with each exhalation?

Interestingly, the relationship between breath and emotion is a two-way street. Each affects as well as reflects the other. We can calm our mind by changing our breathing, and we can change our breathing by calming our mind. It is not uncommon for us to be so wrapped up in ongoing events that we have no awareness of our feelings. We may be operating under extreme anxiety and not even realize it. However, if we learn to monitor our breath periodically we can gain a more accurate insight into our emotional state. Take a look at how you are breathing, then inhale a total breath and make the comparison. Try this exercise several times a day. It will soon become obvious how important the breath is to maintaining your mental equilibrium.

Too often we let our minds interfere with our productivity. At times we find that it takes hours to complete a task that should have taken us no more than fifteen minutes. The frustration drains our energy, leaving us tired and on the verge of falling asleep. These symptoms usually indicate an underoxygenation of the body, especially the brain. Our brain thrives on oxygen. But because of gravity, the blood has to work much harder to make its oxygen delivery above the heart. If our circulation is impaired by lack of exercise or improper breathing, chances are that the brain will not be receiving its maximum supply of oxygen. Our thinking then becomes illogical, and we become moody, cranky and unproductive. Our muscles begin to stagnate with unremoved toxins. In general, we feel as if we are totally useless, unable to accomplish even the simplest task. Such confusion is especially common among sedentary workers who, because of their limited movement, tend to exist in an underoxygenated state.

The *scoop breath* will stretch the muscles and lower the head so that it can become easily suffused with a generous supply of fresh blood. You will return to work with an entirely different attitude, a new sense of perception and an awakened and well-stretched body.

■ SCOOP BREATH

1. Stand with your legs about two feet apart.
2. Slowly raise your hands up over your head as you inhale the total breath.
3. Holding the breath with your arms still raised, bend back as far as possible, giving the spine a good stretch.
4. Still holding the breath, clasp both hands and bend all

the way forward, bringing your hands between your legs. Try to bring your head down to knee level. Now exhale the breath in a series of sniffs rather than full exhalations. With each sniff exhalation, thrust your hands as far back between your legs as possible. If your inhalation has been full, it should take about five or six good sniffs to empty the lungs.

5. Start your next inhalation with your head lowered at knee level.

6. Again bring your arms slowly up over your head as you breathe in the total breath.

7. Bend backward, retaining the breath, and repeat the sniffing exhalation.

The scoop breath should be repeated five times. If done slowly, it gives the blood time to recirculate and reoxygenate. You will feel enhanced mental clarity at the end of this exercise. A similar breath that also stimulates the oxygen supply to the brain is the *expansion breath.*

■ EXPANSION BREATH

1. Standing, spread your legs as far apart as possible.

2. Exhale and bend forward from the waist, letting your head and arms dangle to the floor.

3. As you inhale, keep your hands slightly cupped and bring the arms out from the sides as if you were spreading your wings. Lift the arms until they are level with your shoulders.

4. Hold the breath for a count of ten. Now look up straight ahead and hold the head in that position for a count of three. Then let it fall toward the ground.

5. Slowly let your arms down as you fully exhale.

6. Without lifting your head or standing back up, repeat the exercise ten more times.

7. After the last exhalation let your head dangle for a few more seconds and *slowly* begin to stand back up.

8. Once you are standing erect, take a long, deep inhalation, hold for two or three seconds, exhale and return to work.

When we are intensely involved with a project we often find ourselves becoming weary to the point that words begin to escape our grasp and everything begins to look the same. The *soothing breath* is a short recharging exercise that wipes away the mental confusion that prevents us from concentrating.

■ SOOTHING BREATH

1. Using the fingertips of your left hand, rub the palm of your right hand in a clockwise direction as if you were rubbing a smooth stone. Do this twenty times. Then turn the right hand over and rub the back of the hand for twenty times.
2. Reverse hands and rub the palm of the left hand with your right hand twenty times. Again, turn the hand over and rub its back twenty times.
3. Now place the tips of your fingers gently over your closed eyelids, slightly pressing in. Your palms should cup your cheeks. See Fig. 25.
4. Inhale the total breath.
5. Retain for ten counts.
6. Exhale.
7. Repeat the entire exercise two more times.

By rubbing the hands you stimulate the circulation of your hands, creating a slight warmth or tingling sensation. This is a soothing as well as a revitalizing energy that stills the mind for clearer thought. In another version of this exercise, the hands may be placed one next to the other on the back of your neck after they have been thoroughly rubbed. This should then be followed by three more deep breaths.

■ STRESS

Up until recently, one of the underlying philosophies of our culture has been to push for more, harder and faster. The results have been devastating. The toll has been taken in

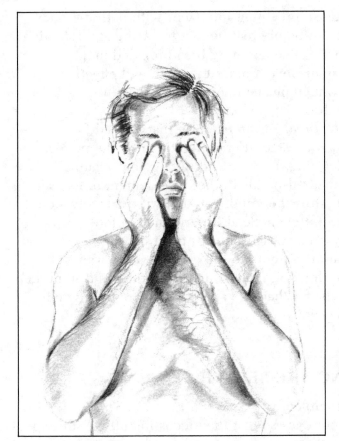

Fig. 25. The Soothing Breath, Step 3. To relax, gently press the eyelids with the fingertips.

lives and physical damage that ranges from heart attacks and ulcers to increased blood pressure and nervous breakdowns. We have come to realize that getting hopelessly anxious and tense only makes our actions less effective and less productive. It is best to keep our body working at a steady, even pace.

We forget that we alone are the ones who are creating this internal physical and mental stress. Therefore we turn to outside sources of help such as various therapies and mood-altering drugs to relieve our stress and strain. Unfortunately they can only provide partial and symptomatic relief. These therapies act more like a temporary Band-Aid, covering up our anxieties rather than actually relieving them. Sedatives can only run interference between ourselves and our problems for so long before the drugs and the problems catch up with us. Because breathing interfaces with both the body and the mind it can be of great benefit to easing and relieving the anxiety of both. By combining breathing and mental relaxation we can achieve a more thorough and effective degree of stress maintenance than we can through dependence on drugs.

Watching the breath is an exercise that is used for bringing on a tranquil state. For meditators it is the perfect prelude before closing the eyes and saying your mantra. Watching the breath also aids in the development of focused concentration. It stills the mind, yet keeps it extremely alert. This exercise is quite beneficial if performed before undertaking any project that requires great concentration and should be repeated at any time the concentration wanes. It helps clarify the thinking process and frees the mind from the useless mental chatter that prevents us from controlling our thoughts and decisions.

■ WATCHING THE BREATH

1. Exhale completely.
2. Lower your eyes so that they focus intently on the tip of your nose. Your eyes may become a little "crossed" as you do. This is fine.
3. Very slowly and gently begin to inhale. You should feel the breath entering at the tip of the nose. This sensation should continue straight up the nose and into the top of the forehead. Even though you feel the stomach inflating and the ribs expanding, keep your attention focused just at the entranceway to the nostrils.
4. When you complete the inhalation, hold the breath for ten counts, which should be based on the pulse beat you feel just under your eyes or in your forehead.
5. Let the exhalation just quietly stream out the end of the nostrils. At the end of each exhalation you may wish to close your eyes for just a moment and let the waves of calmness wash through your entire head.
6. Then begin the next inhalation.

Watching the breath should be done while sitting in a comfortable chair, with your hands in your lap. Because it has such powerful effects on the brain, the exercise should be performed only three times at first. Later you may wish to work your way slowly up to ten repetitions, but this should come only after a month of practice. If you wish continually to enhance the benefits from watching the breath you will want gradually to prolong the length of each inhalation and exhalation. For instilling tranquility and alert relaxation, watching the breath far surpasses a week at the ocean.

The *calming breath* uses the breath and the mind to create a calming sensation throughout the body. The exercise should be used when our tension becomes so severe as to interfere with our normal functioning. It requires the use of the imagination and the mind.

■ CALMING BREATH

1. With your right hand outstretched, fold down the second and third fingers into your palm so that your thumb, ring finger and little finger remain standing.

2. Close your eyes. Place your right thumb against the right nostril, pressing it closed. Slowly begin to inhale the total breath. As you begin to inhale through the left nostril direct the air in a smooth stream straight up to your forehead. Close your eyes and imagine that you are breathing in not just plain air but a very special air that is tinted with a calming color. This may be white, blue, clear or yellow. As the inhalation fills your body, let the color fill the body as well, bringing relaxation, strength and harmony to all parts of the body.

3. At the end of the inhalation, clamp the left nostril shut with the fourth and fifth fingers of the right hand. Hold the breath and the colored air for ten counts. During this time imagine the air gathering up all the tension and anxiety from the body and the one thousand and one unnecessary thoughts from the mind and consolidating them so that they may be expelled all at once with the exhalation.

4. Now, keeping the left nostril closed, release the thumb that is holding the right nostril.

5. The color of the exhalation will be dirtier than that of the inhalation. This exhalation will carry out all the tensions and toxins that the inhalation has accumulated. For example, if you inhaled a calming light-blue breath, the exhalation will be a muddy dark-blue breath.

6. Repeat the entire breath, only this time reverse the procedure by clamping the left nostril with your fourth and fifth fingers and inhaling through the right nostril. The exhalation will be through the left nostril with the right nostril held shut by the thumb. Again, you will inhale your preferred color breath, hold and exhale. Repeat the entire breath four or five times or until the exhalation is the same color as the inhalation.

By focusing on a relaxing and pleasing color we still the mind and give it a chance to locate and expel all the tension from the various parts of the body. Then we exhale them all in one concentrated breath. It may take several repetitions before the exhalation becomes the color of the inhalation. There is nothing you can do to speed up the change of color; it will do so of its own accord, and when it does you will feel entirely different. Over a period of time, your selected color may change. This is fine. Colors are composed of specific frequencies that can affect one's emotional and physical well-being. We all know that blue can relax us, while red can excite us. The color you instinctively choose is most likely of a frequency that is needed by the body. As your needs change, so too will the color of your inhalation change as well.

Because the moment-to-moment functioning of the brain is so interconnected with a healthy supply of oxygen, the possibility exists that the failure of memory in later years is connected with the undernourishment of the brain cells by oxygen. As we age and exercise less, our breathing becomes more shallow. Thus over a period of time circulation is gradually decreased. As the brain receives less and less oxygen certain areas enter dormancy, a kind of suspended animation. Of the little oxygen supplied to the brain, most of it is required for routine functioning. Such luxuries as memory or logical thinking receive only secondary rations of oxygen.

One of the quickest ways to refuel the oxygen in your brain is the *chair bend breath.* It takes less than a minute and can be performed periodically whenever you feel the need for additional oxygen or clearing the mind.

■ CHAIR BEND BREATH

1. Sitting in your chair, exhale completely and bend over. Let your head dangle as close to the floor as possible. Your palms should be touching the floor.
2. Close your eyes and let the blood flow to your head. Stay in this position for a count of fifteen. You may breathe normally while in this position.
3. Slowly lift yourself up and begin to inhale the total breath.
4. As you reach your normal sitting position, exhale. Repeat if desired.

■ FEAR

During fear breathing becomes quick and shallow, irregular or almost arrested. In every monster movie the victim is always heard wheezing quickly and unevenly just before the attack. Rapid-fire breathing only continues to reinforce the anxiety and tremors that accompany fear. It is practically impossible to be afraid once we have regained slow and normal respiration. If we can catch our breathing before it runs away with itself we can quickly reorient our thinking and begin to handle the situation with greater logic and control than if we continue to pant like a dog being chased by a lion.

If you are suddenly startled and your breathing becomes quick and shallow, chances are you'll never be able to handle the situation. Your body will probably freeze from fear. Take a few seconds out and acknowledge to yourself that, yes, you are afraid, but don't let the fear escalate beyond this momentary acknowledgment of its existence. You can shake and shiver all you want, but get that breathing calmed down immediately. Within seconds of controlling your breathing your perception of the situation will change radically and you will be able to handle yourself and the situation with greater control. In *breathing for fear,* the emphasis should be on the inhalation, making it as slow and even as possible.

■ BREATHING FOR FEAR

1. Slowly inhale the total breath, making sure the breath is smooth and steady. By controlling the inhalation you can prevent your body from shaking or becoming immobilized. As you inhale, give yourself the necessary support and confidence by saying, "I can handle this situation."
2. Exhale slowly and evenly. The important step here is slowing down the respiratory rate, yet getting adequate amounts of oxygen into the system as quickly as possible. Just that first long inhalation can do quite a bit for stopping the full range of symptoms that accompany fear. Keep the breath under control and you will be able to act with logic and without fear.

As you continue to explore your body and mind you will find that you can separate yourself from your emotions and problems through breathing. Your perspective of who you are will change a great deal. You will feel yourself developing a stable core of being that is always there. This is who you really are. All that other stuff—fear, pain or anxiety—is just window dressing or stage scenery. As you gain personal control, you will realize that all of these emotions can be changed into positive, constructive emotions. All you have to do is acknowledge to yourself that there are these thoughts in your mind that make you afraid or uncomfortable; but they are nothing more than thoughts, and they can be changed. This is why breathing is so important in these situations. It changes your focus of the situation. After a few breaths you will usually find the situation to be not as intense as you initially imagined. Through time and practice you will be less under the influence of negative emotions and more in control of the workings of your own mind.

Depression appears to be reaching epidemic proportions throughout the country. Many chronically depressed individuals are treated by temporary and cosmetic measures such as Valium to alleviate their sense of despair. Depression can be caused by a million and one different factors. Depression tends to make us sedentary both in terms of action and thought. It is nearly impossible to be thoroughly engaged in some activity and remain depressed. One of the most sought-after benefits of exercise such as jogging is its ability to release depression through physical exertion. As with other negative emotions, you must change the focus of your energies. Most people simply wait for a depression to lift. This passiveness can reinforce the depression and may cause it to linger. Try to catch the depression in its formative stages. Get your mind away from the situation that is making you uncomfortable and passive. The purpose of proper breathing during depression is to reactivate and cleanse both the body and the mind.

■ FORWARD BREATH

1. Stand up and clasp your hands behind your back. Let them rest against the buttocks.
2. Inhale the total breath.
3. Leaning slightly forward, lift your hands up and away from the buttocks as high as they will go. See Fig. 26.
4. With all your strength, forcefully exhale through an open mouth.
5. Return to standing position, inhale and again bend forward, lift your arms and exhale through the mouth in a mighty huff.
6. Repeat ten times.

■ FORWARD BREATH II

1. Stand up and clasp your hands behind your neck.
2. Inhale the total breath.
3. Bend forward from the waist and blow the air out from your mouth. The bending should be done quickly. Try to get your head as far down as possible, hopefully touching your knees.

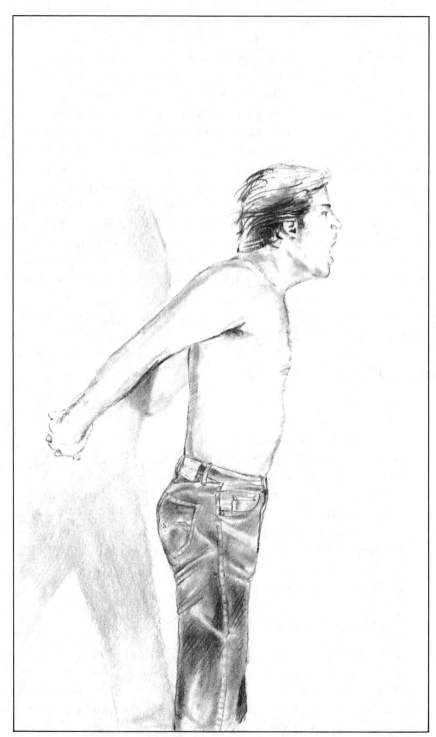

Fig. 26. Forward Breath, Step 3. Lift your hands as high as they will go to stretch the upper back. Exhale through a wide-open mouth.

4. Return to your standing position, inhale and repeat ten times.

Despite the fact that we are rapidly heading into the twenty-first century, we are still using a brain that was created thousands and thousands of years ago. Thus we are still equipped with very primal needs and desires. With our supersonic pace of life we all need to get away from ourselves for brief amounts of time in order to rest from the pressures. For most of us such relaxation is an impossibility. Our minds are constantly focused on the present and working on the future. We have surrounded ourselves with enormous amounts of information and sensory input and the idea of just drifting away from it all seems to be an impossibility. For centuries, music has always had an inspiring and calming effect on our minds and bodies. When music is coupled with breathing we can easily slip into a wonderful dream state for as long as necessary.

■ MUSIC BREATHING

1. Put on a favorite tape or record, preferably one without words that is relaxing in nature.
2. Lie down on your back and close your eyes.
3. Listen to the music for a few minutes, become absorbed in its rhythm.
4. Now begin to breathe through the nose along with the music. There is no specific breathing pattern you should follow. Your breath should be free-form, letting it just move along with the tempo of the music. Although soft jazz or classical music is of course preferable, many people seem perfectly capable of relaxing with the beat of disco. Choose whatever music you feel most comfortable with. The important thing is to let the music create the rhythm of your breath. You should release any control you have over your thoughts or body to the tempo of the music. You can perform this exercise for as long as you feel it necessary.

12 AWARENESS PROGRAM

THE AWARENESS PROGRAM combines breathing with various mental exercises that will bring you in touch with your mental processes and your body. Many of the exercises will stimulate your imagination and allow you to experiment with various mental possibilities. Through these exercises you will become more aware of how your body works and its interaction with your mind, giving you greater mental flexibility. Several of the exercises allow you to see yourself from an entirely different perspective. In this way you gain better insight into who you are, how you do things and what you want.

With inner exploration we can better control and extend our senses. Part of the purpose of the awareness breathing program is to reorient your perceptions of yourself and the exterior world. The *vapor breath* is one of the most pleasant and most relaxing of all breathing exercises. Its purpose is gently to increase your inner sensitivity.

■ VAPOR BREATH

1. In a quiet room, lie on your back on the floor. Hold this position for a minute with your eyes closed. Slowly begin to inhale, inflating the lower abdomen and diaphragm first, then expanding the rib area and finally filling the upper chest. As you inhale, slowly lift your arms so that they rise up and form an arc over you, then keep moving them up and back until they come to rest on the floor behind you. While forming this arc, let your outstretched fingers guide your arms, which should more or less be in line with your outstretched legs. Let the breath enter in a line straight up into your forehead. Check your inhalation, making sure that the breath is silent. If you are making a wheezing noise or a sniffing noise you are breathing in too much too soon. Refine your breath so that it enters the nostrils as if it were a long silken thread, not a gush of wind. Concentrate on the quality of the air you are inhaling. As you inhale, visualize in your mind's eye that this air is a gentle white mist entering your body.

2. Now, with your arms fully extended over your head and your lungs filled with air, hold your breath for as long as comfortably possible. While you are holding your breath you will feel gently rhythmic waves passing over your body. Simultaneously your body will feel as if it is sinking deeper and deeper into the floor. Just let yourself go. You will feel lighter and lighter as the exercise continues.

3. When you feel that it is time to begin the exhalation, keep your eyes closed and slowly begin to raise your outstretched hands off the floor, bringing them up over your head, keeping the fingers pointed straight out the entire time, until the hands come to rest at your sides as you finish the exhalation. Again, let your fingers guide the hands. Visualize the breath you are exhaling as a white mist. Let it slowly envelop you like a cloud of vapors from dry ice. The cloud will begin at your toes and, as you continue to exhale slowly, work its way up until it has surrounded your entire body. At this point just let yourself go and continue to breathe deeply, slowly and normally for another minute or two. Your body will feel incredibly relaxed and almost invisible. Even with your eyes closed you will feel calmly alert. The body may feel as if it is slightly floating an inch or two above the floor in this white mist. Let yourself become more and more absorbed into the cloud. Repeat the entire exercise three or four more times. After the last exhalation just keep your eyes closed until you are ready to open them. During this time you may find yourself dreaming or "sleeping," with a profusion of images floating before your eyes. Upon awakening, you may wonder where you are or where you've been. The relaxation here is deeper than most forms of meditation.

You can use the vapor breath to gain insight into a difficulty or a question you might be considering. As you start the exercise, ask the question in the simplest form possible. The answer that will come to you may appear as an image or from a voice you have never heard before. With the second inhalation, ask the question once again and continue the exercise two more times. At the end of the last exhalation just let your arms rest by your sides as usual. Oftentimes the answer will come during this rest period. The breathing cycle helps clear away much of the mental clutter and confusion that often blocks us from making clear, definitive decisions, and it allows us to become more in touch with our intuitive selves.

Another method for gaining insight into our inner processes is the *lock breath*. This breath closes off all our external sensory organs. The eyes, ears, nose and mouth are completely shut while we hold our breath and explore our internal workings. The lock breath is best done while you are lying down, but you may do it while sitting in a chair. During the exercise you will feel as if you are inside a darkened vacuum of space floating inside your body. There will be no outside noise or light. After a few seconds you will hear your heart beating and your blood pulsing. By slightly pressing down the eyelids you may stimulate the optic nerves, and you will see patterns of color. With the lock breath you can still the outside world long enough to gain entrance to your internal world.

■ LOCK BREATH

1. Inhale the total breath and hold.

2. Now, lock your sensory equipment. Place each thumb over the openings of the ears, sealing out all sound. Next, place each of your second fingers over the bottom of the eyelid, just above the eyelashes. Then with your third fingers, press closed your nostrils. Finally close your lips shut with both ring fingers and pinkies. See Fig. 27.

3. Hold the breath for as long as you feel comfortable.

4. By gently pressing your eyelids with the second fingers you will stimulate your internal visual optic nerves.

5. Keeping your eyes closed, release your fingers. Exhale and then repeat the entire exercise as many times as you like.

Because the mind and body are so interconnected by the breath, breathing can be used to reorient our thinking and sensations away from the outside world and toward our own inner being. The *mind breath* puts the body and mind into a very focused, quiet, meditative state.

■ MIND BREATH

1. Close your eyes and focus them toward the bridge of your nose. Slowly inhale the total breath for ten counts. Breathe in a refined fashion. The breath should silently enter and leave the nose.

2. Hold for twenty counts. During this retention let the body and mind become quiet and still.

3. Slowly exhale for ten counts.

4. Repeat this breath ten times. Afterward you may wish to keep your eyes closed for several minutes and use this

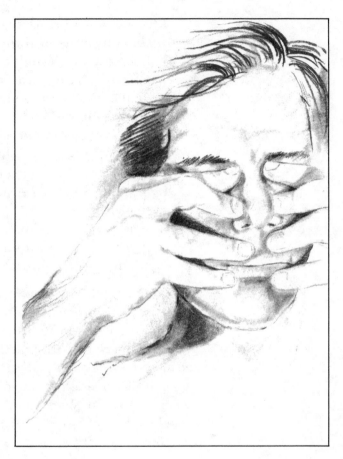

Fig. 27. Lock Breath, Step 2. Close your ears with your thumbs, your eyes with your second fingers, your nose with your third fingers and your lips with your ring fingers on top and your pinkies on bottom.

time to examine your own thoughts or to even keep the mind pleasantly empty.

The purpose of the *healing breath* is to bring your awareness to all parts of the body. Whenever you feel vaguely out of sorts, lie down and practice the healing breath. Aside from mentally re-energizing the body, you will find that your mental check-up can often help you avoid illness.

■ HEALING BREATH

1. Lie down, close your eyes and breathe the mind breath ten times. This will put your body in a quietly alert state.

2. Now, begin breathing the total breath very slowly. Let the breath set its own rhythm.

3. Keeping your eyes closed, mentally begin to look over your body. Starting with the feet, move up the legs, the torso, the arms until you reach the head area. As you mentally scan the body, imagine a stream of white light starting at the feet and making its way through the entire body. Further imagine this stream of light bringing good health and vitality to every part of your body.

4. If you happen to be sick, concentrate the light on that particular area.

5. When you have finished this process, continue to lie with your eyes closed until you feel it is time to arise. Continue the total breath throughout the exercise.

The *information breath* will increase your perceptions of other people. By practicing this breath you will learn to make more intuitive observations and become aware of other people's thinking. With practice you may find yourself second-guessing their statements. This exercise is very good for "getting outside of yourself" whenever you feel too locked in by your own thoughts. By experiencing the thoughts of another person you may give yourself some valuable perspective.

■ INFORMATION BREATH

1. Sitting down, close your eyes and slowly inhale the total breath for ten counts.

2. Hold the breath for twenty counts. Visualize the head of a person you would like to contact. This may be a neighbor, a celebrity or a friend. Quieting your mind, slip their head over yours as if it were a mask. For the rest of the exercise forget your own thoughts and concentrate only on your breathing. Now, imagine you are the other person and see what they are thinking. Just observe them as if you are watching a movie. You may ask the borrowed head questions and watch for its response.

3. After twenty counts, exhale for ten counts.

4. Until you have gotten all the information you wish, continue to breathe in the following pattern. Inhale ten counts. Hold for twenty counts and exhale for ten counts. When you are finished, exhale, then return the person's head and begin your own thinking process. You may now open your eyes.

Throughout our lives we are all faced with difficult decisions—whether or not to buy a house, whom we should marry or where we should go to school. Sometimes we become so confused that making any sort of logical decision becomes virtually impossible. Seeking out the opinions of friends can often help but more often than not will only cloud the issue. What we need is a way to examine all of the alternatives logically and objectively. The *vision breath* sets up a mental laboratory where you can experiment and analyze the possibilities.

■ VISION BREATH

1. Sitting comfortably in a chair, close your eyes. Imagine that on the inside of your forehead is a large television or movie screen.
2. Slowly inhale the total breath for ten counts. Aim the breath to the very center of the forehead.
3. Hold for ten counts.
4. Exhale for ten counts.
5. Continue this rhythm of breathing. As you do so mentally picture on the television screen the event in question. If, for example, you aren't sure about which job to take, picture yourself walking into the office, talking to the boss, working during the day and going home. Notice how you feel, if any problems arise, whether or not you are happy. It is not necessary to try to control the picture on the screen; it will take care of itself.
6. When the film ends, keep your eyes closed for another minute. If you wish you may take a look at another situation or review the one you just saw.

Doctors and designers are aware that color can affect our

mood and sense of well-being. If we walk into a beige room we feel relaxed, light and airy, whereas if we walk into a room that is painted in dark tones we may feel cozy or even slightly depressed. Using color in our environment and our clothing, we can have greater control over our moods. Color can also be incorporated into breathing to help soothe the mind and relax the body. Imagine a pleasant color that you like and visualize this color surrounding you. As you breathe in, inhale the color and let it penetrate every part of your body, bringing tranquility and vitality. By combining the visualization of color with breathing, you give the mind a chance to relax and become focused on just pure color rather than scattered thoughts. The following exercise can be used as a form of soothing meditation.

■ COLOR BREATHING

1. Sit comfortably in a chair with your eyes closed.
2. Exhale completely.
3. Select the color that you desire to inhale. Visualize the air tinted with this color. Deeply inhale the total breath. If, for example, you are inhaling green, you may see yourself sitting surrounded by the most beautiful shade of green. As you inhale, visualize this green entering every nook and crevice of your body, bringing radiant color to your entire body.
4. Hold the breath for ten counts. Let yourself become dissolved in the colored mist that now surrounds your body and is also being held within.
5. Slowly exhale through rounded lips.
6. Repeat three times.

If you do not feel you would like to pick a color to breathe, then just close your eyes before the exercise begins and let a color come to you. That may be just the color you need to work with at that time.

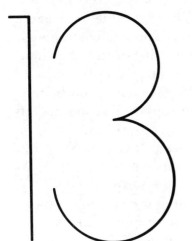

SURVIVAL PROGRAM

THERE ARE MANY emergency situations in which knowing how to control your breathing pattern can mean the difference between life and death. Often in these dire situations people panic; they begin to breathe fast and hard, which requires a great deal of physical energy but does not deliver sufficient oxygen and ultimately works against their survival. Whenever you find yourself suddenly in a situation beyond your control, remember that giving in to panic will not save your life. But more than likely staying calm will. Whether your boat has capsized or you are trapped in an elevator, the first thing you should do is inhale the total breath, hold for a few seconds, exhale and then assess the situation. Chances are, if you use your breath properly you will be able to save yourself or at least keep yourself alive until rescue appears. The emergency breathing techniques can often give an extra margin for survival in the most extreme emergencies.

Although not a common occurrence, entrapment within a confined space does happen. You may get caught in an elevator, a closet or a safe. Situations such as these usually require external help for rescue, but there is a great deal to insure your safety during the wait. The first thing to realize is that you are on a limited budget of air. Through controlled breathing you can economically stretch the air to last as long as possible. The absolute worst thing you can do is jump around, scream and pound on the door, which would be the quickest way to deplete your oxygen supply. Tension, anxiety and panic, though hard to avoid, run a close second for reducing the amount of available oxygen. It cannot be emphasized enough that staying calm means staying alive. As soon as it becomes apparent that you are locked in and trapped, give yourself one good calming breath. Inhale the total breath, hold it for five seconds and exhale with a sigh out of an open mouth. Now begin to survey your predicament. See what, if anything, you can do to escape. Is there an emergency-door release, a telephone or buzzer that can signal help? Is it posssible to slip some paper or fabric under the door as a signal? Is there another exit?

After you have done your best to investigate your surroundings, the next priority is to begin conserving oxygen. Excessive body movement, anxiety and irregular breathing all require substantial amounts of air. To conserve both physical activity and air, the best thing you can do is lie down on the floor. Make yourself comfortable. Because of the confined space you cannot afford to allow a build-up of carbon dioxide in your system which could impair your judgment. For this reason the total breath is the breath of choice. However, in order to economize on your intake of air yet receive good oxygenation, you should refine the breath as you breathe. Instead of sucking in large amounts of air with each inhalation, slow down your rate of respiration. Inhale the air in a very gentle stream rather than a gush. As you refine your inhalation you will feel the air traveling straight up to the forehead and to the back of the head and then down into the lungs. Your inhalations and exhalations should be so smooth that you cannot even hear them. The exhalations should be through the nose and not the mouth. Pause for about ten counts between each breath. By breathing in this manner you will be keeping the body calm and alert and with a good supply of oxygen.

In your signal for help, a loud whistle will utilize your oxygen supply more effectively than frantic yelling and screaming. Surprisingly, few people know how to give out a good strong whistle. If you are trapped in an emergency situation you may wish to alternate a call for help with a whistle.

■ WHISTLING

1. Place the tips of your second fingers together as if to form a triangular space between your hands.
2. Bend your tongue backward as far as it will go. Then place your paired second fingers just on the tip of the tongue. Close your lips tightly around your fingers.
3. Inhale the total breath through your nose. Forcefully exhale over your fingers through the slight opening of the mouth. Adjust the position of your fingers until you get a sharp piercing whistle.

Being trapped in a confined space or lost in the middle of a wilderness, you may find yourself without food and water. In either case you need sustenance to keep the body alive. In these situations it is important to know how to keep your hunger and thirst in check so that your mind does not become fixated on starvation to the exclusion of more practical thoughts. Through specific breaths it is possible to satisfy those needs and "feed" the body.

■ THIRST BREATH I

1. Fold the tip of the tongue back and place it on the roof of the mouth.
2. Close the teeth and form the lips into a grin.
3. Through the mouth suck in the total breath. See Fig. 28.
4. Hold for ten seconds.
5. Exhale through the nose.
6. Repeat three times.

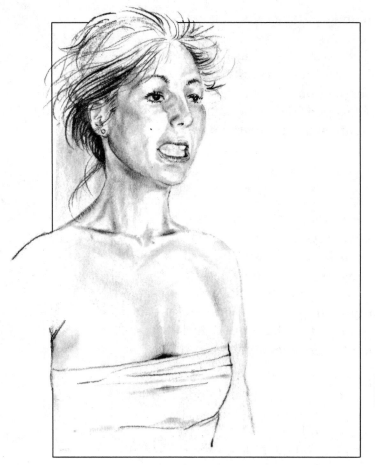

Fig. 28. Thirst Breath I, Step 3.
Form your lips into a grin and
inhale.

■ THIRST BREATH II

1. Smile and place your upper teeth over the lower lip.
2. Through the mouth suck in a total breath.
3. Hold for ten seconds.
4. Exhale through the nose.
5. Repeat three times.

If either variation of the thirst breath is practiced once or twice an hour, you can ward off that dry feeling of thirst while at the same time satisfying the body's need for moisture.

Not being able to eat is not as serious as not being able to breathe. One can go several weeks without food without serious consequences. It is the first day or two that the hunger pains become distracting. After that, one begins to have increased energy and vitality without food. There are methods for getting air into the stomach which fill the stomach and ward off feelings of hunger.

■ FASTING BREATH I

1. Inhale just a sniff through the nostrils.
2. Open the mouth and quickly gulp in a mouthful of air. Close the mouth and swallow the air.
3. Repeat this gulping of air through the mouth until the lungs are full.
4. Exhale through the nose.
5. Repeat three times.

■ FASTING BREATH II

1. Place your teeth together, open the lips in a smile and suck in a mouthful of air.
2. Close the lips. Swallow the air and, just as it begins heading toward the stomach, exhale through the nose.
3. Repeat three times.

If by chance you should be stranded in a snowstorm or get locked in a walk-in freezer, the *fire breath* should keep you warm. By heating up the gastric area and rapidly increasing circulation you can control uncomfortable feelings of extreme cold.

■ FIRE BREATH

1. Sitting down in a cross-legged position with your hands on your thighs; inhale the total breath.
2. Leaning slightly forward from the waist up, forcefully squeeze out the breath by contracting the lower stomach.
3. Release the stomach and then let the air rush back in. The resulting vacuum will create the next inhalation.
4. Again, force the breath out by contracting the lower stomach.

5. To really heat up the body, quicken the rate of inhalation/exhalation. Your breath should sound like a train coming down the tracks. After fifty rapid inhalations stop and slowly inhale the total breath. You will feel the heat generating upward from your stomach to all parts of the body.

One of the best-known methods of emergency breathing measures is artificial respiration. Yet despite massive educational programs very few people possess this skill for saving another's life. Mouth-to-mouth resuscitation is commonly applied to drowning and shock victims but can be employed any time there is a stoppage of breath.

■ ARTIFICIAL RESPIRATION

The person should be lying on his or her back. Tilt the head back as far as possible. If you suspect choking, open the mouth with one hand and with the other, search for any material or food that might be obstructing the airways. If such blockage is present, pull it out. In order to keep the head tilted backward you may have to place one hand under the neck. If the person's mouth is closed, pry it open with your free hand. You are now ready to administer artificial respiration.

■ MOUTH-TO-MOUTH RESPIRATION

1. With your free hand, close the person's nose with your thumb and index finger.
2. Inhale the total breath. Open your mouth wide and fit it over the person's mouth. Blow into the person's mouth with sufficient force to inflate the lungs.
3. After a full exhalation, remove your mouth and let the person's chest fall and exhale.
4. Repeat about every five seconds.

Under certain conditions the person's mouth may be so tightly locked or injured that it is impossible to pry open. At this time, mouth-to-nose resuscitation is as effective as mouth-to-mouth.

■ MOUTH-TO-NOSE RESPIRATION

1. Again, tilt back the person's head and place one hand under the neck to support it. Place the other hand under the chin to hold the jaw and lips closed.
2. Inhale the total breath. Place your lips around the person's nose and blow in to inflate the lungs.
3. Remove your mouth and let the person exhale.
4. If the person is unable to exhale, rotate the head slightly or if possible pry open the mouth and press gently on the chest.
5. Repeat about every five seconds.

Well over two thousand people a year die because of choking. Choking is one of the silliest ways in the world to die just because we took too big a bite from a sandwich or because we tried to eat, drink and talk all at the same time. Most chokers panic, which increases their asphyxiation and paralysis. If someone is choking, your first attempt should be to open his or her mouth, search around for the food and remove it. If you can't find the blockage, have the person raise his hands high over his head, close his mouth, press his tongue firmly against the roof of his mouth and slowly breathe in through the nose.

For any number of reasons we may find ourselves afloat in the ocean miles from shore and without a life vest. Maybe our boat capsized, the plane crashed or our scuba gear failed. There are ways to inflate the lungs so that they function as a life preserver, keeping us safely afloat until help arrives. Like an inner tube, the lungs, once filled with air, can provide lifesaving buoyancy.

■ FLOATING AND BREATHING

1. First of all, manage through some simple stroking of the arms and kicking of the feet to get yourself to the water's surface.
2. With your arms stretched out to either side, lift your nose out of the water and fill your lungs about three quarters full of air.
3. Continually treading water is tiring; it is best just to

let the lungs support you for the next several seconds. While holding your breath you may wish to take a fetal position. Your head will be down in the water with your back curved and your arms and legs just hanging.

4. To take another breath, blow the air out through the mouth, bringing your arms out to the side for one stroke and have your legs give a little kick.

5. Now lift your head so that it is above the water, breathe in and return to your floating fetal position. Try to expend as little energy as is necssary in movement. Concentrate on just comfortably floating. As you give that stroke toward the surface for a breath, direct that stroke toward the direction of the shore.

Children often hold their parents ransom for new bicycles and such by threatening to hold their breath until they die. Showing natural concern for the health and safety of the child, parents often quickly give in and promise anything if the child will only start breathing again. Of course this reinforces these terrorist tactics, and it won't be long before the parent is obeying the child's every command with each new threat of self-asphyxiation. The seemingly defenseless parent who is at the mercy of the child's threat does have one major trump card at his or her disposal—the infinite intelligence of the body. When we hold our breath we quickly begin to starve the body of its necessary oxygen supply, but the body is not one to be hijacked. Once the carbon dioxide reaches dangerous concentrations, the breath holder will pass out and in the state of unconsciousness will automatically start breathing again. The parent's only concern during this breathing ransom is that the fainting child is not in a position to fall and crack his or her head. So let your kid hold his breath for as long as he likes; just make sure that he's sitting in a well-upholstered chair.

Some people react to emotional or environmental stress by breathing at quicker rates. Their breathing may become like the panting of a dog. This is called hyperventilation. During hyperventilation the body becomes superoxygenated and the normal oxygen/carbon dioxide ratio is radically imbalanced. Once the blood becomes so saturated with excess oxygen the person may feel dizzy and faint, and the breathing may slow down or even stop for a brief period of time. In such cases the body will eventually re-establish its normal oxygen/carbon dioxide ratio. However, you can greatly speed up the body's recovery rate by having the hyperventilator breathe into a paper bag for a minute or two. Place the bag over his mouth and nose and just let him rebreathe his own air. This will quickly boost the level of carbon dioxide in the bloodstream, returning it to normal.

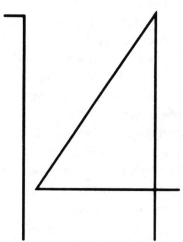

AFTERWORD: BREATHING FOR LIFE

By consciously applying the breath to nearly every aspect of your daily life, from sports and health to mental clarity and tranquility, you begin to exercise greater control over the workings of your own body and mind. This step toward greater self-sufficiency will penetrate every aspect of your life. No longer are you so susceptible to physical complaints such as colds, lack of energy or headaches. No longer do your emotions run away with themselves, resulting in chronic tension or insomnia. The point is that *total breathing* is one of the most important keys to your total well-being.

Now that you have experienced all types of breathing for various circumstances, the most important thing is to use it. Although these exercises were designed for specific needs, they may be expanded to your individual use. For example, if you suddenly find yourself tense and can't remember the exact directions for a calming breath, then begin with the total breath. From there, guide your breathing into a pattern that will relax you.

As you go through the various programs in the book you will be training your breath automatically to react to your emotions, your actions and your environment. Throughout the day you will suddenly find yourself changing the way you breathe to get more oxygen into the body just as your energy level begins to drop or as your tension level begins to build.

The most important aspect of the entire total breathing program is to use it constantly. Become aware of your breathing and use it to its fullest advantage. It takes but a second to rearrange your breathing. Your body will let you know when you have to change your breathing. It won't be necessary to take a breath check every ten minutes.

As good breathing becomes more ingrained with your way of life, you will find it to be one of your more enjoyable activities. The rewards of total breathing are certainly worth the small investment of time and practice. Total breathing can and will accomplish for your body and mind what no other exercise or training program can—the ability to physiologically control and influence your vitality, your emotions and your well-being.

Catalog

If you are interested in a list of fine Paperback
books, covering a wide range of subjects
and interests, send your name and address,
requesting your free catalog, to:

McGraw-Hill Paperbacks
1221 Avenue of Americas
New York, N.Y. 10020